"*Lie There And Lose Weight* arrived this n[...] there. It's charming, intelligent, persona[...] pointers in the read. I like best of all that i[...] and no lectures! In a world of endless weig[...] that speaks a personal truth and perhaps there may be some truth in it for me... and you too." — **CCH Pounder**

"**Insightful**, endearing and surprisingly funny...." — *The Brooklyn Daily Eagle*

"**A slender volume that will definitely make your volume slender.**" — *New York Times* best-selling author Peter David.

"**No one hates to lose more than John Ordover**. So you can imagine my surprise when he lost 100 pounds without breaking a sweat.... Amazing!" –*New York Times* best-selling author David Mack

"**Losing weight is hard for everyone**, but few can write about it with as much warmth, humor and honesty as John Ordover does in this remarkable book. He takes us along as he loses more than a hundred pounds, relating every step of his journey with refreshing candor and insight. His experience should serve as an inspiration to anyone looking to lose weight and keep it off." – **David K. Randall,** *New York Times* **bestselling author of** *Dreamland: Adventures in the Strange Science of Sleep.*

"**With elegant grace and a touch of humor**, John Ordover takes us through his fight to lose 100 pounds. The portrait of his struggle and celebration of his success will motivate of anyone looking to shed pounds. Let this book be your guide on how you, too, can lie there and lose weight. — **Thomas A. McKean, author of** *Soon Will Come the Light: A View From Inside the Autism Puzzle*

"*Lie There and Lose Weight*...**reads like a thrilling suspense story** that plays out one pound at a time, as John Ordover takes us through his struggle not only to lose weight but to save his life. An inspiring, must have book for everyone who finds losing weight to be a real pain in the a**." — *New York Times* **bestselling author Diane Carey**

"**What I admire most about** *Lie There and Lose Weight* is that it doesn't contain the phrase 'made easy.' John Ordover acknowledges that losing weight — and keeping it off — is incredibly difficult and very hard work. Bravo."—-**Keith R.A. DeCandido, best-selling author of** *Star Trek: The Klingon Art of War*

"**The best weight loss book I have ever read.** So much of what John Ordover writes I have experienced, felt and dealt with. That my son has autism means taking care of myself is mandatory, so I can be around to take care of him. Fifteen months ago I was in the best shape of my life. Now I'm dealing with major physical issues, gained 25 pounds, and am wanting my old body and clothes back. I was feeling the futility of it all and was buoyed ... by learning I could lose weight without running a 5K 3 times a week." — **Becky Large, Champion Autism Network."**

"**This book has already helped me lose 50 pounds!**" — Warren Lapine, Publisher Wilder Publications.

Lie There and Lose Weight

How I Lost 100 Pounds By Doing Next to Nothing

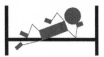

Wilder Publications, Inc.
PO Box 632
Floyd VA 24091

Hard Cover ISBN 13: 978-1-5154-1933-4
Trade Paper ISBN 13: 978-1-5154-1934-1

Lie There and Lose Weight

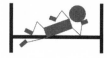

How I Lost 100 Pounds By Doing Next to Nothing

by John J. Ordover

To my wife, Carol Greenburg, my love and inspiration, without whom nothing is possible; and to our son, Arren Isaac Ordover, for whom everything is possible.

Table of Contents

Introduction

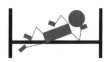

On October 13th, 2015, I set myself the goal of losing 100 pounds and keeping it off. This was after years of going up or down 50, 60, 70 pounds and reaching my highest weight at 305.6 pounds. It took me a year to lose those pounds, and it was tough going every single day of that year. It is tough now keeping it off.

Losing weight, no matter what any book, magazine article, or television commercial says is an incredibly difficult thing. Along the way I learned a few tricks and figured out others that helped me take the edge off, which I'll share here, but there is nothing I know of that can make losing weight easy or fun. I'm sharing what I thought and felt as I lost weight in the hope that it will be of some help to others trying to do the same thing.

I documented my struggle starting on October 13th, 2015, on the Facebook Social Network Service. The support and advice I got from my Facebook friends was instrumental in my being able to get through this challenge and right on through to today. Male or female, there is so much shame connected to being fat in our society. Going public with my weight struggle was hard but it helped immensely.

Interacting with other people with the same struggles or who are professionals in this area also taught me what I needed to do to succeed, and I'm sharing that here as best I can.

That there was always someone on Facebook willing to listen if I wanted to complain, or who agreed to reward me in various non-monetary but significant ways for making certain goals, was wonderful. So this book is in part a compilation of my Facebook posts over that year (and a bit more) and includes some quotes from my Facebook friends as well. I thank them for allowing me to include their encouraging words.

What I'm Not Going To Do

October 13, 2015
Week 0: 305.6 pounds
Starting new weight loss program. Goal is to lose 100 pounds then see where I stand.

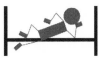

Anyone who knows me, heck, anyone who has ever met me or heard me speak, would expect my writing a book that is entirely about me to be not only easy for me but inevitable. I love to talk about myself, love to be the center of attention, I'm quite loud and quite talkative. If it seems I'm the kind of guy whose favorite topic of conversation is himself, that conclusion is quite probably correct.

Nevertheless it turns out writing entirely about my own physical and emotional experiences, really letting people behind the wall, is a struggle. I'd much rather go with my naturally bossy nature and just tell people what to do. It's far easier to point out other people's flaws and challenges than it is to take a hard look at my own. It's a lot more fun to tell other people what to do than to do it myself. Despite the self-restraint required I will not be telling people what to do in this book.

That said, here's the one thing you must do: consult your doctor before starting any weight-loss plan. See how easily that comes to me?

Here's what I'm really not going to do:

I'm not going to tell you what diet you should be on. Any diet that restricts calories will work as well as any other and it is likely you already have all the information you need to go on a diet. Anything that worked for you before will likely work again. The challenge is sticking to it.

I'm not going to provide you with recipes, or limit your food choices, or tell you to adopt one program or another. While Weight Watchers worked well for me, nothing in this book is drawn from their program, and no advice I give is under their direction. Any opinions I express in this book, living or dead, are not necessarily something Weight Watchers endorses or agrees with.

I'm not going to use euphemistic terms like "lifestyle change." Minimizing my struggle with euphemisms didn't work for me. For me a diet by any other name was still a diet and calling it a lifestyle change wouldn't have made it any less unpleasant. Plus, I wasn't "heavy-set" or "overweight" or even "obese." I was fat.

I'm not going to tell you I had gastric bypass surgery because I didn't, although I'm often asked if I did.

I'm not going to try to sell you anything, or rather anything other than this book which you already bought, or at least someone did, or you wouldn't be reading it. Or maybe you stole it, in which case shame on you.

In a country with more fat people per acre than any other, everyone who struggles to lose weight feels entirely alone. At least when we're not looking out of the corner of our eye and thinking "that guy's fatter than I'll ever be!" only to wake up a year later fatter than that guy and scanning for someone even fatter.

What I am hoping to do by baring my inner self on these pages is connect with the isolated fat person who feels imprisoned, limited, or undeserving of love: you are not alone, you are not unloved, you are not less than human.

Getting Fat

October 20, 2015
Week 1 of my new weight-loss plan: lost 2.4 lbs. At that rate, only 41.6 weeks left
to go.

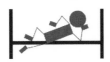

So how fat was I? I topped off at 305.6 pounds but numbers don't really paint a picture. I am 5'11" tall with a normal frame. At 300 pounds plus I wasn't stuck in my house or anything, and fit through doorways, but I was certainly fat enough people seeing me walk down the street would think, and sometimes say, "look at that fat guy, how'd he let himself get that way?" Or old friends would think or very helpfully say "you've packed on a few pounds, I see" or other such comments. I recall being singled out as a funeral broke up by someone pointing at me from not as far across the room as they thought and saying "Well, John probably knows all the good places to eat." Charming comments like that. I fit in theater seats but only barely, in airline seats I needed a seatbelt extender. So how'd I get that way?

Getting fat was not a goal I set when I was 14 (until then I had been average-to-skinny) but something that came with adolescence. Pounds came with the pimples. The appetite of a pubescent boy is legendary, and when mine came on it came on hard. I went from a skinny nerdy kid to a fat nerdy kid in one year. From my point of view I was only eating when I was hungry and only as much as I wanted to eat (more on that later) but pow, I was growing out as well as up. Doing that for forty years, with only short breaks for temporary weight loss programs, was what got me to three-hundred-and-five-point-six pounds.

Clearly something was wrong.

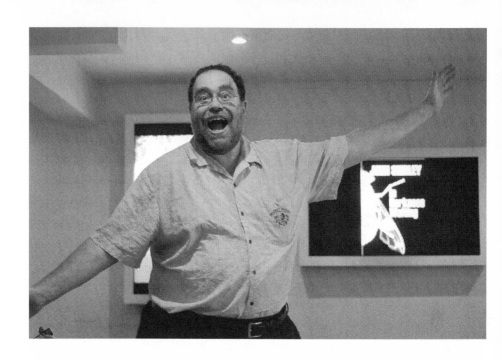

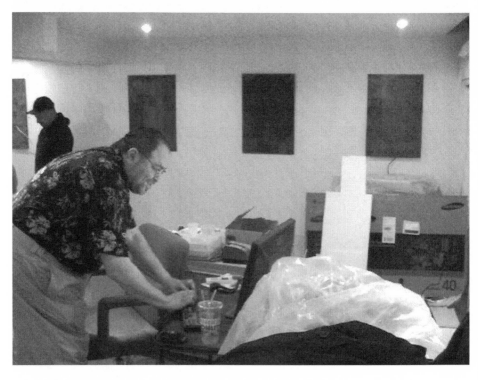

The Hunger Switch

October 27, 2015
Tuesday Weight Loss Report:
I have lost another 3.4 pounds, for a total weight loss of 5.8 pounds over two weeks, leaving me at 299.8. Since my goal is to reach 205, that leaves me another 94.8 pounds to go.

At my current average weight loss of 2.9 pounds per week, that leaves me with another 32.6 weeks to go. I am doing this on a disgustingly healthy diet, so no concerns there.

I am always hungry. I am hungry as I write this. I'm hungry as you are reading it. If I ate an entire pizza, I would be hungry again within thirty minutes. This is simply a fact of my life. What was up with that? Maybe I was hungry because I was stressed or anxious or under pressure or not dealing with a trauma or another psychological situation; maybe I had some kind of poorly understood biological issue. Maybe something like that was behind it all. I didn't know what my issue was and I still don't (and certainly don't know what yours is).

Whatever it was, though, I experienced it all as hunger. Somehow my "hunger switch" was broken, locked into "always on." If I was going to lose weight and keep it off, I was going to have to accept that I was hungry and deal with it some way other than eating.

Doctors and Friends

Nov 3, 2015
Tuesday Weight Loss Report:
I have lost another 1.8 pounds, for a total weight loss of 7.6 pounds over three weeks, leaving me at 298 even. Since my goal is to reach 205, that leaves me another 93 pounds to go.

At my current average weight loss of 2.53 pounds per week, that leaves me with another 36 weeks to go.

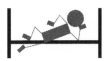

I consulted with three different doctors during my diet: two metabolic specialists and one psychiatrist whom I have been seeing for 25 years off and on. At the height of my weight curve, Dr. David Case laid my options out for me: my health was so at risk at over three hundred pounds, between my blood pressure, my heart rate, cholesterol and all the usual suspects, that I had to seriously consider gastric bypass surgery of one kind or another. I met with a friend who had had the surgery done and he outlined what I would have to do to care for myself after the procedure, and that sounded far worse to me, or at least no better than what I would have to do to lose weight. Plus it is major surgery with a painful recovery period and a huge host of its own risks.

I rejected surgery and told Dr. Case that it wasn't for me (although it was certainly right for my friend), and I have no idea if it would be right for you, dear reader, or not. This time I would lose the weight once and for all. He had expected that response; he had suggested the surgery to drive home the seriousness of my losing weight. I took his point.

The Emotion Explosion

November 10, 2015
Tuesday Weight Loss Report:
I have lost another 2 pounds, for a total weight loss of 9.6 pounds over four weeks, leaving me at 296 even. Since my goal is to reach 205, that leaves me another 91 pounds to go. At my current average weight loss of 2.4 pounds per week, that leaves me with another 38 weeks to go.

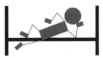

I had several emotional reactions as I started my diet. These were among them:

"Why me?" How come everyone else gets to eat as much as they want and they don't gain weight? The answer is that Hunger Switch I spoke of before. My Hunger Switch is set wrong, and despite all the talk about the mythical "set points" for the body, there is no way to reset it.

"This sucks!" Which I felt because having to diet really does suck. You can pretty it up however you want, but it totally sucks.

"This is really hard!" I felt because it is really hard.

"I don't want to have to do this!" I whined because I didn't want to have to do it.

And so on.

That said, I have a friend with failing kidneys. He goes in for dialysis at least three times a week. He absolutely hates it. Loathes it. Is sometimes in tears about it. But he does it right on time every week because the other option is sickness and an early death. Those same conditions applied to me. I have a teenage son who is autistic and who has limited ability with language. He and my wife need me to be part of their lives as long as I can be. I was free to hate the diet, but I had no choice but to be on it.

Ramblings

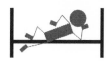

Are there emotional issues that contribute to eating too much? Probably, since emotional issues influence everything we do. What's certain is the emotional battering someone would get if somehow they woke up fat tomorrow. All of the following examples really happened, although not all of them happened to me:

Walking into a room and having everyone look at you, categorize you as beneath them and look away, or look at you with pity.

Declining desert at a restaurant and having the server say "Watching your weight, huh? Good for you honey!" or even worse "Trying to lose weight? It's about time." Or ordering whipped cream on your pancakes and the server saying "You sure you need that, honey, aren't the pancakes enough?" Or putting your plate down at an all-you-can-eat diner and having a stranger next to you say "Be careful, that's how you got so big in the first place!"

Being told by someone you used to have a crush on "Why didn't you tell me you felt that way? Looks aren't that important to me."

Hearing a clerk in a clothing store say "I'm afraid we have nothing in your size!" in a very loud voice, clearly desperate to assure other customers that no one your size shops at their classy establishment.

Someone coming up to you and saying "Where do you get your clothing? I have an aunt almost as big as you are!" Or asking "Is your whole family as big as you?"

Having a friend of the appropriate sex say "I'm so horny I could have sex with anyone!" while you're sitting right there, and when you raise your hand they say "Well, not you of course" since fat people are sexually invisible.

That's just the tip of the iceberg, of course. It gets far worse and I could quote examples all day. I won't speak to what's going on in the minds of the clerks, servers or strangers, but whatever it is Wil Wheaton's "don't be a dick!" comes to mind.

Don't Trust Anyone Under 130 (Pounds)

November 17, 2015
Tuesday Weight Loss Report:
I have lost another 3 pounds, for a total weight loss of 12.6 pounds over five weeks, leaving me at 293 pounds even. Since my goal is to reach 205, that leaves me another 88 pounds to go. At my current average weight loss of 2.5 pounds per week, that leaves me with another 35.2 weeks to go.

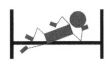

I started my diet while Michelle Obama was still focused on her anti-fatness campaign. It quickly became clear to me that while the then-First-Lady's heart was in the right place, to the best of my knowledge she had never been fat and had never had to lose weight herself. As with many naturally slender people, Ms. Obama was stuck on the idea that people are fat due to a lack of information and lack of exercise. With that in mind, she set out to provide both education on the issue and access to exercise.

Of course it's true that some people don't know which foods have more calories than others, and certainly education on that score doesn't hurt those people even if it is just a reminder. I was not one of those people. As with most fat people, I had been on multiple diets that worked just fine but that I could not sustain. More information was of no use to me. Neither was doing more exercise. It takes an hour of exercise to burn off a handful of peanuts and eating peanuts takes a lot less time and effort than an hour at the gym. If I didn't find a way to stick to a diet, I was lost.

I found that people who are naturally thin had little information of value to impart to me about how to become thinner and a lot of them see their thinness as a sign of superior virtue or psychological vigor. Which it isn't, any more than walking around with healthy kidneys makes someone more noble or moral than someone born with a kidney disorder. It just makes them luckier.

Dieting is Hard; Exercise Makes it Harder

November 24, 2015
Tuesday Weight Loss Report:
I have lost yet another 3 pounds, for a total weight loss of 15.6 pounds over 6 weeks, leaving me at 290 pounds even. Since my goal is to reach 205, that leaves me another 85 pounds to go. At my current average weight loss of 2.6 pounds per week, that leaves me with another 32.7 weeks to go.

I also got my weight watchers 5% Bravo sticker and charm, having lost 5 percent of the body weight I walked in with.

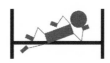

I tried working exercise into my diet a bunch of times, both with and without formal guidance. What I found was that exercise did not help me lose weight, it made losing weight that much harder.

There are a handful of reasons for this that go beyond my expertise so I will say only that exercise makes me hungry. Not just usual hunger but ravenous-panicky-want-to-grab-the-sandwich-out-of-someone-else's-hands hungry. The more I exercised the hungrier I got. So after putting in the work to burn, say, fifty calories, which is a whole lot of exercise, I couldn't keep myself from eating three hundred calories. All in pursuit of the vague goal of "fitness" that I could find no consistent definition for. In the end I decided that for me, dieting to lose weight and exercising were not compatible. Since I was losing weight on a consistent basis without exercising, I decided not to continue. Which sounds like a thoughtful and rational decision but what really happened was exercise was so boring, so unpleasant, and so counter-productive that I just stopped doing it.

Ramblings

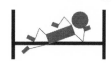

For those who are unmotivated to exercise for many reasons but especially because they, like me, find it dull beyond words, I hereby wish into existence John Ordover's Space Bike. Connected to a video game system, it wouldn't be merely a visual of a road, the point of view would shift as the bike is turned left and right and monsters would pop up. Monsters that could be shot at by pushing buttons on the handle bar and the faster you pedaled, the faster the screen would go by, or any of a thousand variations on that theme.

It really does seem easy to do, and if this book becomes the worldwide bestseller it deserves to be, then maybe someone from a gaming company will read this and reach out to me. Or maybe this book will sell only ten copies but one of those ten people will work at, or know someone who works at, a gaming company.

No, I'm not going back on what I've said about exercise. It is not an important part of losing weight, and I found it actually worked against me. But even I think exercise is a good thing for reasons unrelated to weight loss. Even having lost all that weight, I still find exercising falls somewhere between watching grass grow and watching paint dry as a way to kill an hour, or even twenty minutes. I want the gaming companies to realize there is a huge market out there that is not served well by the current offerings on the Wii or Kinect or any other move-while-you-play system as of this writing.

What the video systems offer seems to be modeled on exercise videos and sports games. How about a fantasy role-playing game that involves having to swing a virtual sword left and right to mow down the monsters, or a secret agent game that involves running and jumping and climbing to escape or fight, or a super-hero game that does the same? Build the exercise into the game-play and you'll make millions. Or as above develop John Ordover's Space Bike, with controls that snap onto an at-home exercycle.

There's good money in doing good. Trust me.

'Fessing Up

I did not post a report. I had gone up by six-tenths of a pound to 290.6 and was still thinking of my posts as "weight loss reports." No weight loss, nothing to report, right?

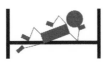

After thinking it over for a few days I decided I had to be honest about what was going on, that if I was going to post about moving forward I had to also post about slipping back. If I was going to lean on people for support I had to trust I would get sympathy when I was struggling, not just praise when I met a goal. I was still a bit nervous about it but reassured myself that hey, it was Facebook, and anyone who was a schmuck to me I could just unfriend or block.

It might be going too far to say that everyone was supportive, but pretty much everyone was and very few people had to be unfriended. It was an important lesson for me.

So when I picked up the posting on the date below, I changed the header to "weight report." It was important that I come clean, in public, when I gained as well as when I lost.

Distraction Reaction

December 8, 2015
Tuesday Weight Report:
I have lost 1.8 pounds since last week, putting me at 288.8 for a total weight loss of 16.8 pounds over 8 weeks. Since my goal is to reach 205, that leaves me another 83.8 pounds to go. At my current average weight loss of 2.02 pounds per week, that leaves me with another 41 weeks to go.

To expand a bit, my weekly target is, and always has been, to be somewhere between 1 and 2 pounds down each week. Having lost 3 lbs a week for a few weeks in a row was nice but not sustainable, as weight loss always slows down.

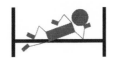

I was hungry the entire time I was losing weight. I tried many different ways to cope but found distractions were the most effective method of sticking with it. Those distractions could be anything from watching TV to playing on Facebook to doing things I was actually supposed to be doing, which I tried to spend as little time doing as possible, but there you have it. The hungrier I was, the more productive I became. Plus an odd thing happened to me. Slowly I found that when I felt hungry, my reflexive reaction to reach for food turned into a reflexive reaction to find something to do that would take my mind off it. I couldn't stop myself from feeling hungry but over time I could change how I reacted to that feeling.

Anything enjoyable could work, from fantasy football to concerts to gardening to collecting stamps or playing cards or mahjong. Paintball, even. Those aren't my things but they're someone's, and there's something out there for everyone. My wife suggests a good distraction for women might be a mani-pedi or other beauty treatments, which reminds me to suggest that for men getting an old-fashioned hot-towel shave, which I am now addicted to, could work.

Think First

December 15, 2015
Tuesday Weight Report:
I have lost 3.4 pounds since last week, putting me at 285.4 for a total weight loss of 20.2 pounds over 9 weeks. Since my goal is to reach 205, that leaves me another 80.4 pounds to go. At my current average weight loss of 2.24 pounds per week, that leaves me with another 36 weeks to go.

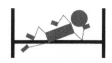

If I sat down in front of the television set with a big bowl of popcorn, chips, or pretty much anything, I would eat reflexively and inattentively until the bowl was empty. Same if I was sitting around with friends chatting and someone put a bowl of Tostitos down in front of me. If I opened a bag of pretzels, even if I swore to myself I would only eat four or five, I would wander into another room, bag in hand, and finish the whole thing. That first handful of whatever snack food you'd care to name shut down my brain and took control of my hand (yes, really) and I would just keep on putting it in my mouth while daydreaming about other things.

I swear snack food has soothing, mind-numbing capacities that could guide us all to ruin, or to peace-on-earth, a roly-poly kind of peace. What to do about this? Well, as Tock explained to Milo in *The Phantom Tollbooth*, "if you got someplace by not thinking the best way to escape from it is by thinking." After some time thinking I realized if I couldn't open a bag or pour a bowl of anything without eating the entire thing, I shouldn't open the bag or pour the bowl in the first place. If I also found it hard not to open the bag, don't bring the bag into the house in the first place. More on that later.

Just Rewards

December 22, 2015
Tuesday Weight and Activity Report:
I have gained .6 pounds since last week, putting me at 286, for a total weight loss of 19.6 pounds over 10 weeks. Since my goal is to reach 205, that leaves me another 81 pounds to go. At my current average weight loss of 2 pounds per week, that leaves me with another 40.5 weeks to go.

On the activity front, for the last week I have been doing 5 miles per day on my recumbent exercise bicycle. This is new, and I have no idea how it may have impacted my weight, but I will keep at it.

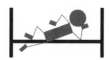

When I felt particularly down, I needed a pick me up. That pick me up had always been picking up food. When I felt like celebrating, I would celebrate with food. When I weighed in and had lost weight, my reflex was to celebrate with the snack I had "earned." If I didn't have that food I felt down, or deprived of a reward I was entitled to, and had no idea how else to celebrate good news. I had to find another approach, because damn it, I had done all my chores, run all my errands, done a lot of boring stuff I didn't want to.

And you know, I did deserve a reward. But that reward didn't have to be food.

The reward could be just about anything else. I started looking around for something else.

I found that I was incredibly easy to please. A fifty-cent plastic slinky was rewarding enough, or any other toy from a gumball machine. So was a magazine. So was seeing a super-hero movie in the middle of the day. So was planning a fishing trip (not even taking one, just carving out the time to plan something I enjoy). Changing what I rewarded myself with was a huge part of how I kept on keeping on.

Salt of the Earth

December 29, 2015
Tuesday Weight and Activity Report:
I have lost 6.6 pounds (yes, six pounds plus six-tenths of a pound) since last week, putting me at 279.4. for a total weight loss of 26.2 pounds over 11 weeks. Since my goal is to reach 205, that leaves me another 74.6 pounds to go. At my current average weight loss of 2.4 pounds per week, that leaves me with another 31 weeks to go.

This extreme weight loss is most likely a result of my cutting back on sodium - salt - over the last week, so I dropped a lot of water-weight. But wherever it came from, I'll take it. :)

On the activity front, doing five miles a day caused my calves to stiffen up and cramp; I am taking a week off, then resuming at 5 miles Monday, Tuesday, and Wednesday, and building up to more miles three times a week so my muscles can grow between sessions.

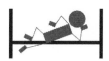

When I told my doctor about the weight loss above he was pissed at me. That amount is way too much for one week, and when I told him it was due to taking sodium out of my diet he exclaimed "I didn't tell you to do that! It can be dangerous!"

And here I thought I was being so good.

"Salt isn't good for you" is another of those things that are pounded into us by pop culture, and yes he told me, there are some conditions, like extremely high blood pressure, that call for a low-salt diet. But cutting out sodium and such risks not only dehydration but destabilizing your heart rate and other bad things I didn't really listen to because that was enough for me. Your doctor might tell you differently, but what my doctor told me was "If your kidneys are functioning, and yours are, quit worrying about salt. Any weight you lose from dropping it is only water anyway."

So I quit quitting salt. I was much happier and more energetic with the salt. I also realized it wasn't cutting out the salt that made a difference, it was cutting out the things we use as excuses to eat salt, like salted nuts and salted pretzels and salted chips and, sadly, cheese, which has far more salt in it than I ever knew. A friend suggested seaweed snacks, a roasted and salted version of the outer wrap on sushi rolls that can be eaten like potato chips. They sounded gross but it turned out I liked them, They satisfy salt cravings and have very few calories..

Lie There and Lose Weight

Jan 5, 2016

I have lost .6 pounds (six-tenths of a pound) since last week, putting me at 278.8, for a total weight loss of 26.8 pounds over 12 weeks. Since my goal is to reach 205, that leaves me another 74 pounds to go. At my current average weight loss of 2.25 pounds per week, that leaves me with another 32.8 weeks to go.

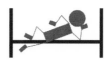

That exercise is the true path to losing weight is something we are bombarded with from all sides. We're told you can't lose weight without it, or that a particular new-fangled piece of exercise equipment being advertised on late-night TV will lead to guaranteed thinness. On top of which if you somehow manage to lose weight by dieting alone, you're told it's impossible to keep it off without exercising.

My experience with exercise, plus discussions with my consultants and my observation of my friends who started diet-and-exercise programs with great fan-fare that they fell off of within a month or two showed me that for me exercise was the wrench in the works, the fly in the ointment, the thing that "everyone knew" you had to do to lose weight that was actually keeping me fat. While it works for some people, it didn't work for me. That exercise is necessary to losing weight is so hard-wired into our society I kept going back to it in fits and starts.

When I dieted and exercised at the same time, I was sending my body two different messages: build up mass (in the form of muscle) while taking off mass (the fat I wanted to get rid of).

Plus it took me twenty minutes or so to burn off a hundred calories, and twenty seconds to put it back on. A few peanuts, a single apple, or a small bag of any snack food and everything I had sweated for was undone. So instead of exercising to speed up weight loss, I just cut another hundred calories out of my diet.

Losing weight and building muscle are two different activities that "everyone knows" are inextricably linked, but separating those two things is what led me to succeed.

Ramblings

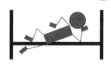

There are a lot of things that float around the diet world as received wisdom that are simply not true or not completely accurate. Some are innocuous, some lead people down a false path, and some (like avoiding salt) can be actively dangerous.

Gluten: unless you have a wheat allergy, celiac syndrome, or some other medically diagnosed condition, there is no reason to avoid gluten. It won't hurt to avoid it but it can be extremely inconvenient, and if the goal is only weight-loss there's no purpose to going gluten-free.

Dairy: less than one percent of people of European and African descent are lactose intolerant or allergic to milk. Without that diagnosis there is no reason to avoid dairy. Even for the lactose intolerant it is not likely to cause you any more trouble than a little gas. If it does a little Lactaid goes a long way.

Sugar: diabetics and hypoglycemics, or people with some other problem relating to blood sugar levels, should of course avoid sugar. Other than having such a condition, there is little reason to avoid sugar. That said, a whole lot of people find that rather than making them feel full, eating something containing sugar makes them hungrier. Everyone has to figure out the sugar thing themselves.

Meat: humans are omnivores, meaning we are made to eat both vegetables and animal flesh. There are those who avoid eating meat for philosophical reasons, and that's fine. Others have had their doctor tell them meat has a bad impact on their health for whatever reason, that's fine too. Otherwise there is absolutely no reason not to eat meat. It's highly satisfying, very tasty, and in controlled portions fine for dieting.

Diet Soda: unless someone reacts badly to one of the ingredients there is no reason for them to avoid diet soda; if diet soda gives them headaches or they don't like the taste or they feel sick after drinking it then of course they should stop drinking it. Word on the street is diet soda will increase hunger. Is that true? There are preliminary studies in fruit flies and mice that imply it might, so fruit flies or mice who want to lose weight should avoid diet soda. Not sure about any other species. For me it was a diet-saver (and fully approved of by my doctor).

To sum up: it took consulting with my doctor and some trial-and-error for me to figure out what worked for me, and the same likely holds for everyone else. No one knows what is right for someone else to eat, and what someone else eats is none of anyone else's business.

The Squash Fiasco

Jan 12, 2016
Tuesday Weight Report:
I have lost 1.2 pounds since last week, putting me at 277.6, for a total weight loss of 28 pounds even over 13 weeks. Since my goal is to reach 205, that leaves me another 72.6 pounds to go. At my current average weight loss of 2.15 pounds per week, that leaves me with another 33.7 weeks to go.

I am very pleased that I lost weight despite having mistakenly added squash to my diet. Back on the right path now. :)

I have lost an average of just over 2 pounds a week, and am quite pleased with my progress. :)

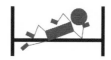

I have a problem with the beyond-me concept of "small amounts." I was allowed "small amounts" of squash of various kinds, primarily zucchini, on the program I was following. So, although I had never particularly liked squash, out of desperation I started using in it recipes and found that properly cooked and seasoned, it was very good. I added more, and more and more, and got a spiralizer, which is a very cool gadget that lets you magically transform a zucchini into a pile of noodle-sized strips that can be used as pasta, and added more, and more.... Turns out zucchini is for me what people call a "trigger food." A food that causes the desire to eat more of it along with any food it's next to or that is in the same room or building. I call those things "shuts-down-my-brain food." When I start eating something on my trigger list, and it's a depressingly long list (everyone has their own list) I stop thinking. Not thinking makes me fatter. When I catch myself eating certain foods unthinkingly, I cut them out of my diet. I'll miss you, squash, we had some good times together, but it's over now. It's not you, it's me.

Tonight at Nine

Jan 19, 2016
Tuesday Weight Report:
I have lost 4 (four) pounds since last week, putting me at 273.6, for a total weight loss of 32 pounds even over 14 weeks. Since my goal is to reach 205, that leaves me another 68.6 pounds to go. At my current average weight loss of 2.29 pounds per week, that leaves me with another 30 weeks to go.

Hitting 32 pounds is a benchmark because that means I have lost more than 10 percent of my initial body weight (305.6 lbs). It also means I get a 10% chip from Weight Watchers for my keyring, where it is sitting happily next to my 5 percent chip from a few weeks ago and my "lost 25 lbs" chip (which is cute, it's a miniature weight like used in a weight room, with 25 lbs stamped on it.

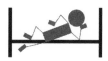

Every night at 9:00 I would find myself eating what I called a "second dinner" or craving one. It might be that Hunger Switch thing, or it might be that my grandmother would always give me a bedtime snack of cookies and milk when I stayed over at her house, or it might be any number of things. The cause didn't matter, I had to deal with the situation, since it was hard to go to sleep hungry.

I coped in a couple of ways. I discovered that while I was hungry at nine, if I held out until ten often the hunger would go away. If it didn't, I would have a small salty snack or a small glass of chicken broth, and either way go to sleep immediately. The only time I could be certain I wasn't going to eat was when I was asleep, and letting myself get too tired was one of the major triggers for hunger. I got into the habit of going to sleep around ten no matter what, leaving me less time awake and hungry.

The Coming of the Benchmarks

Jan 26, 2016
Full Tuesday Weight Report:
I have lost .6 (6/10ths) of a pound since last week, putting me at 273 pounds even, for a total weight loss of 32.6 pounds over 15 weeks. Since my goal is to reach 205, that leaves me another 68 pounds to go. At my current average weight loss of 2.17 pounds per week, that leaves me with another 31.3 weeks to go.
Benchmarks to Come:
33 and 1/3rd pounds, one-third of the way to my goal.
50 pounds, halfway to my goal.
54.6 pounds lost, which will put me where I was 18 months ago.
Thank you all for your support as I work through this unpleasantness!

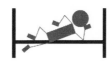

It is hard for me to stick to a long-term goal. I'm better at sprints than marathons. Short-term unpleasantness is less, well, less unpleasant than the long-term version. I decided I would set up intermediate goals so the hundred-pound target, which seemed very far away over many burning coals, wouldn't be the only sense of accomplishment I would get. I needed mileposts along the way to mark achievements as I went. Hence the benchmarks, which will soon multiply greatly from this humble beginning and get closer and closer together.

Where I was 18 Months Earlier

Feb 2, 2016
Tuesday Weight Report:
I have lost 2.6 (two-and-six-tenths) of a pound since last week, putting me at 270.4 pounds, for a total weight loss of 35.2 pounds over 16 weeks. Since my goal is to reach 205, that leaves me another 65.4 pounds to go. At my current average weight loss of 2.2 pounds per week, that leaves me with another 29.7 weeks to go.
Benchmark Achieved:
I am now over 1/3rd of the way to my goal.
Upcoming benchmarks are:
50 pounds lost, halfway to my goal.
54.6 pounds lost, which will put me where I was in August of 2014.
66.6 pounds lost, two-thirds of the way to goal.
75 pounds lost, three-quarters of the way toward my goal.
Thank you all for your support!

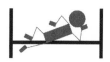

The sharp-eyed reader will have noticed my referring to "where I was in August of 2014" in the benchmarks above. By August of 2014 I had lost fifty pounds from where I had started. Then I was blindsided by an emotional grenade of family issues that I won't detail here and could not maintain the necessary focus. Within a couple of months I had not only gained back everything I had lost but put more on besides, for like the seventeenth time. This time around I was going to make it no matter what life-thing ambushed me, and I was going to keep it off. That meant setting up a support system that would keep me on target no matter what truckload of manure got emptied on me Biff Tannen style.

That's where Weight Watchers and my Facebook friends came through for me. The weekly Weight Watchers meetings were a great place to share whatever came along that would make me likely to fall off the wagon, and no group of people I've met in real life could have possibly been more supportive. Earlier I mentioned how alone everyone trying to lose weight feels, and for me shattering that sense of isolation was vital.

Sleep It Off

February 9, 2016
Tuesday Weight Report:
I have lost 2.0 (two) pounds since last week, putting me at 268.4 pounds, for a total weight loss of 37.2 pounds over 17 weeks. Since my goal is to reach 205, that leaves me another 63.4 pounds to go. At my current average weight loss of 2.3 pounds per week, that leaves me with another 27.5 weeks to go.

Got my 4 Months Weight Watchers trinket today...it's surprising how meaningful those can be. :)

Upcoming Benchmarks are:
50 pounds lost, halfway to my goal.
54.6 pounds lost, which will put me where I was in August of 2014.
66.6 pounds lost, two-thirds of the way to goal.
75 pounds lost, three-quarters of the way toward my goal.
Thank you all for your support!

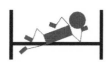

I talked earlier about how important it was for me to get enough sleep. That wasn't just a matter of getting to bed early. It was a matter of recognizing when I was reaching for food when what I really needed was a nap. Between my family and my work and just wanting to have a life sometimes sleep got away from me, and I'd reach for food to perk me up and keep me going. Which it did. But it also kept me from losing weight.

As David K. Randall, author of *Dreamland*, the *New York Times* bestselling book about sleep, put it recently:

"Lack of sleep doesn't just lead to poor decision making, making it more likely for someone to snack on a late night burger and fries. The

body has an innate need for sleep, and reacts to decreased hours of sleep by increasing its demands for carbohydrates and slowing its metabolism, as if out for revenge on the brain that made it become over-tired."

To lose weight I had to re-prioritize, make sleep more important than it had been, and do my best to grab twenty-minute naps whenever I could.

A Matter of Taste

Feb 16, 2016
Tuesday Weight Report:
I have lost 1.8 (one point eight) pounds since last week, putting me at 266.6 pounds, for a total weight loss of 39 pounds over 18 weeks. Since my goal is to reach 205, that leaves me another 61.6 pounds to go. At my current average weight loss of 2.16 pounds per week, that leaves me with another 28.5 weeks to go.

New Benchmarks added:
40 pounds lost: Try on next-size down pants.
Because in general men lose a pants size every 20 pounds down, I try on pants one size down every 20 lb. Also I've reached the last belt-hole on my current belt.

Benchmarks to Come:
40 pounds lost: Try on next-size down pants.
Upcoming benchmarks are:
50 pounds lost, halfway to my goal.
54.6 pounds lost, which will put me where I was in August of 2014.
60 pounds Lost: Try on next-size-down pants.
66.6 pounds lost, two-thirds of the way to goal.
75 pounds lost, three-quarters of the way toward my goal.
80 pounds lost, try on next-size-down pants.
85.6 pounds lost, I will be "Overweight" rather than "Obese."
Thank you all for your support!

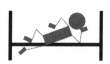

What is hunger anyway? When it comes to food the dictionary definition ranges from "feel like eating now" to "starving to death." The definition I came up with, as I worked on dealing with hunger in other ways than eating was "I am not hungry until things I don't like start to look good." Then I expanded it to the more surprising "I am not hungry until things I don't like start to taste good."

This led to "If I'm spending more than thirty seconds staring into the refrigerator trying to decide what to eat then I am not actually hungry and should close the door and walk away."

As I went along I found that a huge range of foods, from peppers both sweet and hot to cauliflower and cabbage, were suddenly not only palatable but enjoyable. The biggest surprise was suddenly liking spicy food in general, which I had always loathed. I think I was unconsciously sorting food by how many calories it had rather than bothering with taste, with the high-calorie stuff on the top of my favorites list. I'm not certain what really happened but I now appreciate a far greater range of flavors than I did before. Who knew a red pepper could taste better to me than a bag of chips?

Ramblings

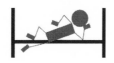

What is hunger? According to the *Farlex and Partners' Medical Dictionary* (2009 edition), hunger is:

"A sensation resulting from lack of food, characterized by a dull or acute pain referred to the epigastrium or lower part of chest. It is usually accompanied by weakness and an overwhelming desire to eat. Hunger pains coincide with powerful contractions of the stomach. Hunger is distinguished from appetite in that hunger is the physical drive to eat, while appetite is the psychological drive to eat. Hunger is affected by the physiological interaction of hormones and hormone-like factors, while appetite is affected by habits, culture, taste, and many other factors."

That really doesn't capture how the desire to eat slowly pushes other thoughts out of my head, and how likely I am to seek food without conscious thought. Which is why I found recognizing the unconscious reflex to eat and finding ways to short-circuit it helped my diet. A lot of my tricks turn out to be similar to techniques used to help people cope with chronic pain, which makes sense because hunger is a lot like a migraine that gets worse throughout the day. What I call a "broken hunger switch" is in the same category and could perhaps be treated with the same methods.

Over and Over Again

Feb 23, 2016

Tuesday Weight Report:

I have lost 3.0 (three-point-zero) pounds since last week, putting me at 263.6 pounds, for a total weight loss of 42 pounds over 19 weeks. Since my goal is to reach 205, that leaves me another 58.6 pounds to go. At my current average weight loss of 2.21 pounds per week, that leaves me with another 26.5 weeks to go.

Benchmark Achieved:

40 pounds lost: Tried on next-size down pants. (which fit). Got 5 lb star from WW. YAY!

Benchmarks to Come:

45 pounds lost: Get 5 lb star from WW.

50 pounds lost, halfway to my goal. 5 lb star from WW, charm from WW.

51 pounds lost, more than halfway to goal.

54.6 pounds lost, which will put me where I was in August of 2014.

55 pounds lost, 5 lb star from WW.

60 pounds lost: Try on next-size-down pants. 5 lb star from WW.

65 pounds lost, 5 lb star from WW.

66.6 pounds lost, two-thirds of the way to goal.

70 pounds lost, 5 lb star from WW.

75 pounds lost, three-quarters of the way toward my goal. 5 lb star from WW.

80 pounds lost, try on next-size-down pants. 5 lb star from WW.

85 pounds lost, 5 lb star from WW.

85.6 pounds lost, I will be "Overweight" rather than "Obese."

90 pounds lost, 5 lb star from WW.

95 pounds lost, 5 lb star from WW.

100 pounds, 5 lb star, 100 lbs charm from WW. Get free lifetime membership in WW.

"Glam" photo shoot in tailored suit.

Thank you all for your support!

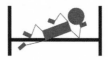

You'll notice I added on a few benchmarks, because I found the more I had, the closer together, and the more immediate the rewards, the better I did. I realized as I reached this stage that society stressed that brilliant insight and sudden genius were respected (I have had my moments) while simply doing the same thing over and over was considered mindless drudgery. Yet piling one stone on another, day after day after day, is how the pyramids were built. It's how every building was built. I quit looking for some kind of epiphany that would suddenly make something that is inherently tedious quick and simple.

It's at least an equally valid process to do the same thing over and over until you've accomplished something grand. For me losing weight was a matter of waking up each day and doing pretty much the same thing I had done the day before. The benchmarks helped a bit with a sense of recognition for doing that, but that's what it was.

Playing the Percentages

March 1, 2016

Tuesday Weight Report:

I have lost 0.8 (zero-point-eight) pounds since last week, putting me at 262.8 pounds, for a total weight loss of 42.8 pounds over 20 weeks. Since my goal is to reach 205, that leaves me another 57.6 pounds to go. At my current average weight loss of 2.14 pounds per week, that leaves me with another 26.9 weeks to go.

I've noticed as I go through this that the week after I lose 3 pounds or more I lose substantially less the next week or even gain some. That's why what I look at is the average weight lost per week. It's been over 2 pounds a week on average for quite a while, which is the level I hope to maintain. I will post my weekly stats separately for those of you who are into such things.

Benchmarks to Come:

45 pounds lost: Get 5 lb star from WW.

50 pounds lost, halfway to my goal. 5 lb star from WW, charm from WW.

51 pounds lost, more than halfway to goal.

54.6 pounds lost, which will put me where I was in August of 2014.

55 pounds lost, 5 lb star from WW.

60 pounds lost: Try on next-size-down pants.

65 pounds lost, 5 lb star from WW.

66.6 pounds lost, two-thirds of the way to goal.

70 pounds lost, 5 lb star from WW.

75 pounds lost, three-quarters of the way toward my goal. 5 lb star from WW.

80 pounds lost, try on next-size-down pants. 5 lb star from WW.

85 pounds lost, 5 lb star from WW.

85.6 pounds lost, I will be "Overweight" rather than "Obese."

90 pounds lost, 5 lb star from WW.

95 pounds lost, 5 lb star from WW.

100 pounds, 5 lb star, 100 lbs charm from WW. Get free lifetime membership in WW.

"Glam" photo shoot in tailored suit.

Thank you all for your support!

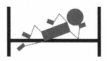

One of the great things about losing a set amount of weight is that how much each pound counts toward the final goal goes up with each lost pound. To clarify, I set out to lose a hundred pounds. The first ten pounds dropped ten percent of my target weight loss, and left me 90 pounds to go. The next ten pounds, with 80 pounds to go, dropped 11 percent of my remaining goal, up from ten. The next ten I dropped, leaving me at 70, was just over twelve percent of my remaining goal, and so on. What this meant for me, physically and emotionally, is that it felt like the weight loss was getting faster. Remember, my goal wasn't to weigh zero pounds, it was to weigh 205.6. So it felt like my weight loss was speeding up even though it wasn't. In fact, it was about to slow down.

What Was It?

March 8, 2016

Tuesday Weight Report:

I have once again lost 0.8 (zero-point-eight) pounds since last week, putting me at 262.00 pounds, for a total weight loss of 43.6 pounds over 21 weeks. Since my goal is to reach 205, that leaves me another 56.8 pounds to go. At my current average weight loss of 2.08 pounds per week, that leaves me with another 25.2 weeks to go.

I had hoped to lose more, and I may make some adjustments to my diet, but as long as my average weekly weight loss stays above 1.5 lbs I'm satisfied.

Benchmarks to Come:

45 pounds lost: Get 5 lb star from WW.

50 pounds lost, halfway to my goal. 5 lb star from WW, charm from WW.

51 pounds lost, more than halfway to goal.

54.6 pounds lost, which will put me where I was in August of 2014.

55 pounds lost, 5 lb star from WW.

60 pounds lost: Try on next-size-down pants.

65 pounds lost, 5 lb star from WW.

66.6 pounds lost, two-thirds of the way to goal.

70 pounds lost, 5 lb star from WW.

75 pounds lost, three-quarters of the way toward my goal. 5 lb star from WW.

80 pounds lost, try on next-size-down pants. 5 lb star from WW.

85 pounds lost, 5 lb star from WW.

85.6 pounds lost, I will be "Overweight" rather than "Obese."

90 pounds lost, 5 lb star from WW.

95 pounds lost, 5 lb star from WW.

100 pounds, 5 lb star, 100 lbs charm from WW. Get free lifetime membership in WW.

"Glam" photo shoot in tailored suit.

Thank you all for your support!

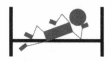

I was extremely frustrated at this point. Two weeks with no significant weight loss was something new, especially when I didn't have re-hydration or being sloppy with my diet to explain it. It was time to check with my doctor and see what was what. He said bluntly "When this happens, drop your calories twenty percent and keep on going." Not good news, because dropping calories meant cutting my portion size which was already, compared to the way I had been eating, pretty puny. But I did it. I took twenty percent off the amount I was eating at every meal.

It was rough. After feeling like I had adapted nicely and wasn't quite so hungry as I had been, here I was, suddenly hungry again. I realized the way to tell I was losing weight was if I felt hungry. Just no way around that. So I ramped up my coping mechanisms, distraction and non-food rewards, and as one of my Facebook friends said, "embraced the suck." It would be a couple of months before I found out just why it sucked so much and why I had to cut calories to jump start my weight loss.

A Big Pot Of...

March 15, 2016
Tuesday Weight Report:
I have lost 3.6 (three-point-six) pounds since last week, putting me at 258.4 pounds, for a total weight loss of 47.2 pounds over 22 weeks. Since my goal is to reach 205, that leaves me another 52.8 pounds to go. At my current average weight loss of 2.14 pounds per week, that leaves me with another 24.6 weeks to go.
Benchmark Achieved:
45 pounds lost: Got 5 lb star from WW.
Benchmarks to Come:
50 pounds lost, halfway to my goal. 5 lb star from WW, charm from WW.
51 pounds lost, more than halfway to goal.
54.6 pounds lost, which will put me where I was in August of 2014.
55 pounds lost, 5 lb star from WW.
60 pounds lost: Try on next-size-down pants.
65 pounds lost, 5 lb star from WW.
66.6 pounds lost, two-thirds of the way to goal.
70 pounds lost, 5 lb star from WW.
75 pounds lost, three-quarters of the way toward my goal. 5 lb star from WW.
80 pounds lost, try on next-size-down pants. 5 lb star from WW.
85 pounds lost, 5 lb star from WW.
85.6 pounds lost, I will be "Overweight" rather than "Obese."
90 pounds lost, 5 lb star from WW.
95 pounds lost, 5 lb star from WW.
100 pounds, 5 lb star, 100 lbs charm from WW. Get free lifetime membership in WW.
"Glam" photo shoot in tailored suit.
Thank you all for your support!

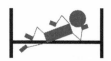

As I went along this process I was shocked to discover that some people find the idea of eating leftovers disgusting. I can't connect to that at all. Anything that was good the first day tastes even better the second day, at least to me. This technique will not work for the leftover averse.

I figured out what I could eat on my diet, in what size portions, then made a big pot of it. Then for each meal for the few days it would last all I would have to do to stay on my plan is scoop out the amount my diet limited me to. Yes, it got boring, but making my next meal boring helped me stay on track. If it got too boring I would just make another big pot of something else on my diet, or even two, and alternate meals. Making the easiest thing to grab out of the fridge always the right thing to eat made everything easier.

The Biggest Loser

March 22, 2016
Tuesday Weight Report:
I have lost 3.0 (three-point-zero) pounds since last week, putting me at 255.4 pounds, for a total weight loss of 50.2 pounds over 23 weeks. Since my goal is to reach 205, that leaves me another 50.4 pounds to go. At my current average weight loss of 2.18 pounds per week, that leaves me with another 23.1 weeks to go.
Benchmark Achieved:
50 pounds lost, halfway to my goal. 5 lb star from WW, 50 lb lost charm from WW.
Benchmarks to Come:
51 pounds lost, more than halfway to goal.
54.6 pounds lost, which will put me where I was in August of 2014.
55 pounds lost, 5 lb star from WW.
60 pounds lost: Try on next-size-down pants.
65 pounds lost, 5 lb star from WW.
66.6 pounds lost, two-thirds of the way to goal.
70 pounds lost, 5 lb star from WW.
75 pounds lost, three-quarters of the way toward my goal. 5 lb star from WW, 75 lbs lost charm from WW.
80 pounds lost, try on next-size-down pants. 5 lb star from WW.
85 pounds lost, 5 lb star from WW.
85.6 pounds lost, I will be "Overweight" rather than "Obese."
90 pounds lost, 5 lb star from WW.
95 pounds lost, 5 lb star from WW.
100 pounds, 5 lb star, 100 lbs charm from WW. Get free lifetime membership in WW.
"Glam" photo shoot in tailored suit.
Thank you all for your support!

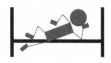

So in the middle of my diet the New York Times prints an article about the TV show The Biggest Loser. It was quite popular for a while. The contestants on the show were fat people who were put through a grueling diet-and-exercise program and the winner was the one who had lost the largest amount of weight. The article was about how after the show and the forced program was over, all the contestants had regained their initial weight and were at least as fat now as they were before or more.

The article said this result meant that losing weight and keeping it off created some kind of metabolic change that made it impossible to keep the weight off. There is nothing more discouraging than the "newspaper of record" telling someone fighting the fat that it was a pointless and inherently losing battle. The next day, however, the Times printed this:

To the Editor:

Your article on the metabolic rate of "The Biggest Loser" contestants raises serious concerns about drawing broad conclusions from fourteen individuals undergoing an extreme and unsustainable regimen. The National Institutes of Health study reported a considerable drop in the metabolic rate of contestants, despite a weight regain, on average, of more than two-thirds of the original pounds lost.

In contrast, my colleagues and I have published two larger studies showing almost no negative effect of weight loss on metabolism. In one study, 145 participants lost 11 percent of their weight and experienced a drop in metabolic rate of just 5 percent and a decrease in calorie requirements of 7 percent.

In another study, of 30 gastric bypass patients, weight loss was 38 percent and caused a decrease in metabolic rate of 26 percent and a decrease in total calorie requirements of 24 percent. Far from documenting adverse metabolic efficiency, these studies demonstrated a healthy parallel decrease in weight, metabolism and calorie needs.

Data from "The Biggest Loser" should not be extrapolated beyond the effects of extreme and unsustainable diets that are not recommended for general use.

SUSAN B. ROBERTS

Boston

The writer is director of the Energy Metabolism Laboratory and a professor of nutrition at Tufts University.

This letter brought Dr. Susan Roberts to my attention. I emailed her, not just to thank her for her letter countering The Biggest Loser article, but to ask her professional opinion on why my weight loss had dropped off despite staying to the same diet, and why I had had to cut calories twenty percent to start the weight loss again.

Here's what she wrote back:

"If you lose let's say 30% of your weight your calorie requirements will be about 30% lower when you finish, it's a proportional change."

So that was the secret behind the leveling out of weight loss called "a plateau." The more weight I lost, the fewer calories my body burned. I would shrink only until I'd balance out again, at which time I would stop losing weight unless I cut calories, meaning portions, down yet again. Another thing about losing weight that sucked: the more weight I lost, the less I got to eat. It also cemented in my mind what I had thought from the beginning: there would be no Before and After. It would all come down to Then and Now.

Then and Now

March 29, 2016

Tuesday Weight Report:

I have lost 2.8 (two-point-eight) pounds since last week, putting me at 252.6 lbs, for a total weight loss of 53 pounds over 24 weeks. Since my goal is to reach 205, that leaves me another 47.6 pounds to go. At my current average weight loss of 2.2 pounds per week, that leaves me with another 21.6 weeks to go

Benchmark Achieved:

Over 51 pounds lost, more than halfway to goal.

Benchmarks to Come:

54.6 pounds lost, which will put me where I was in August of 2014.

55 pounds lost, 5 lb star from WW.

60 pounds lost: Try on next-size-down pants. 5 lb star from WW.

65 pounds lost, 5 lb star from WW.

66.6 pounds lost, two-thirds of the way to goal.

70 pounds lost, 5 lb star from WW.

75 pounds lost, three-quarters of the way toward my goal. 5 lb star from WW, 75 lbs lost charm from WW.

80 pounds lost, try on next-size-down pants. 5 lb star from WW.

85 pounds lost, 5 lb star from WW.

85.6 pounds lost, I will be "Overweight" rather than "Obese."

90 pounds lost, 5 lb star from WW.

95 pounds lost, 5 lb star from WW.

100 pounds, 5 lb star, 100 lbs charm from WW. Get free lifetime membership in WW.

"Glam" photo shoot in tailored suit.

Thank you all for your support!

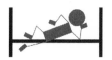

Before and After photos are mandatory in any book about weight loss (see pages 16 and 152). Before, the model or author is Fat; After, they are Thin. This creates the idea that there is an end in sight, that there will be some point in time after which all worries about weight are over with. Maybe that is true for some people, but it most certainly is not true for me. For me there is only Then, when I was fat, and Now, when I am at my target weight. Here in the Now portion of my life, I still have to think carefully before I eat, and if I take my eye off the ball, my weight shoots right back up. To this day I have to weigh in weekly and if I don't my weight goes up again. It goes up even if I do weigh in, but with weekly feedback I can adjust what I'm doing when I'm only one or two pounds up, not ten or twenty pounds up. For me, being overweight is a chronic condition that needs constant attention, and yeah, it's a pain-in-the-ass. But I'm here, and if I want to stay here, that's what I have to do.

Just Throw it Out

April 5, 2016
Tuesday Weight Report:
I have lost 2.6 (two-point-six) pounds since last week, putting me at 250.0 lbs, for a total weight loss of 55.6 pounds over 25 weeks. Since my goal is to reach 205, that leaves me another 45.0 pounds to go. At my current average weight loss of 2.2 pounds per week, that leaves me with another 20.4 weeks to go.
Benchmarks Achieved:
54.6 pounds lost, which will put me where I was in August of 2014; also 55 pounds lost, 5 lb star from WW.

This is particularly significant to me, because in 2013 I was 299 pounds, but by summer of 2014 I had lost 48 pounds, putting me at 251 pounds. I then had an emotional bomb dropped on me and wound up regaining all the weight I had lost and more, putting me at 305.6 pounds. So until this week, I had been regaining lost ground, or re-losing previously lost pounds, or however you want to put it. By hitting 250 pounds, I have moved one pound into new territory. So yay me. :)
Benchmarks to Come:
60 pounds lost: Try on next-size-down pants.
65 pounds lost, 5 lb star from WW.
66.6 pounds lost, two-thirds of the way to goal.
70 pounds lost, 5 lb star from WW.
75 pounds lost, three-quarters of the way toward my goal. 5 lb star from WW, 75 lbs lost charm from WW.
80 pounds lost, try on next-size-down pants. 5 lb star from WW.
85 pounds lost, 5 lb star from WW.
85.6 pounds lost, I will be "Overweight" rather than "Obese."
90 pounds lost, 5 lb star from WW.
95 pounds lost, 5 lb star from WW.

100 pounds, 5 lb star, 100 lbs charm from WW. Get free lifetime membership in WW.

"Glam" photo shoot in tailored suit.

Thank you all for your support!

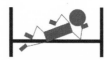

To many people it is a sin to waste food, and I feel that myself. There are people all over who aren't getting enough to eat from day to day and throwing away perfectly good food rather than eating it seems horrible even to those of us living in well-fed societies. So how could I cope when a second (or third) helping is just too hard to resist?

One option was knocking on a neighbor's door and saying "I'm trying to lose weight and I need help. Please take the rest of this lasagna off my hands so I don't eat it." Never had a bad reaction to that, never got a "No, thank you!" People were completely sympathetic to my situation and as far as I can tell everyone likes getting surprise food. Other options I looked into were donating some kinds of food to a nearby shelter soup kitchen or aide center, or finding a hospital or gas station or any place that is open all night, a convenience store maybe, and dropping my leftovers off with them. I found there is usually someone nearby who would be happy to get a treat.

That said, if there is absolutely no other option, if putting it in the fridge for "later" meant that "later" would come that same evening, I threw it away. I felt bad about doing that, but it was better than eating it.

This works for me at the candy counter too. Sometimes I simply can't resist buying something that's wrong for me. It may have something to do with my needing to feel rewarded, I don't know. Once I'd bought it, I found that I could then give it to someone else or throw it away. Yeah, buying it and throwing it away was a waste of money. It would be worse, though, for me to have spent the money and then eaten the candy.

The Ineffable Lightness of Thinning

April 12, 2016
Tuesday Weight Report:
I have lost 2.0 (two-point-zero) pounds since last week, putting me at 248.0 lbs, for a total weight loss of 57.6 pounds over 26 weeks. Since my goal is to reach 205, that leaves me another 42.4 pounds to go. At my current average weight loss of 2.2 pounds per week, that leaves me with another 19.2 weeks to go.
Benchmarks to Come:
60 pounds lost: Try on next-size-down pants. Get 5 lb star from WW.
65 pounds lost, 5 lb star from WW.
66.6 pounds lost, 239 pounds, two-thirds of the way to goal and into the 230s.
70 pounds lost, 5 lb star from WW.
75 pounds lost, three-quarters of the way toward my goal. 5 lb star from WW, 75 lbs lost charm from WW.
76.6 pounds lost, weight at 229, and into the 220s.
80 pounds lost, try on next-size-down pants. 5 lb star from WW.
85 pounds lost, 5 lb star from WW.
85.6 pounds lost, I will be "Overweight" rather than "Obese."
86.6 pounds lost, weight 219, so in the 210s.
90 pounds lost, 5 lb star from WW.
95 pounds lost, 5 lb star from WW.
96.6 pounds lost, weight 209, so in the 200s.
100 pounds, 5 lb star, 100 lbs charm from WW. Get free lifetime membership in WW.
"Glam" photo shoot in tailored suit.
Thank you all for your support!

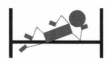

I get asked quite often how it feels to be thinner. It feels great. It's like living on a lighter-gravity planet, every step feels like it's going to take me bounding across the Earth. Distances seem much shorter. When I was a hundred pounds heavier, ten blocks seemed like a long way to walk; now a mile seems easily doable. It is also now possible for me to dress reasonably well, to walk into a random men's store and get a suit or other ensemble.

One of the reasons I dressed poorly when I was fat was because it isn't that easy to dress well. Buying clothing was a very demoralizing and isolating experience. I had to go to a euphemistically named "big and tall" store, where the clothing is vastly more expensive and there are very few options. Everyone shopping there is avoiding each other's gaze. It wasn't quite hell but it wasn't any fun either. So being more in the middle of the size range is very pleasant and is one of my motivations to keep my weight-loss on track.

Restricted eating and the underlying hunger that goes along with it remain unpleasant, although further advice from Dr. Roberts about which foods were most likely to stem hunger the longest helped greatly (more details can be found in her book *The "I" Diet* and its associated website www.theidiet.com). I also found that I had been relying on my fat stomach to hold myself upright so my back muscles were very weak, leading to strains and inflammation that I am still dealing with. But even with that, it's a hell of a lot better than being fat.

SABOTAGE!

April 19, 2016

Tuesday Weight Report:

I have lost 2.8 (two-point-eight) pounds since last week, putting me at 245.2 lbs, for a total weight loss of 60.4 pounds over 27 weeks. Since my goal is to reach 205, that leaves me another 40.2 pounds to go. At my current average weight loss of 2.2 pounds per week, that leaves me with another 18.2 weeks to go.

Listed Benchmarks Achieved:

60 pounds lost: Tried on next-size-down pants (which fit perfectly). Got 12th 5 lb star from WW.

Upcoming Benchmarks:

65 pounds lost, 5 lb star from WW.

66.6 pounds lost, 239 pounds, two-thirds of the way to goal and into the 230s.

70 pounds lost, 5 lb star from WW.

75 pounds lost, three-quarters of the way toward my goal. 5 lb star from WW, 75 lbs lost charm from WW.

76.6 pounds lost, weight at 229, and into the 220s.

80 pounds lost, try on next-size-down pants. 5 lb star from WW.

85 pounds lost, 5 lb star from WW.

85.6 pounds lost, I will be "Overweight" rather than "Obese."

86.6 pounds lost, weight 219, so in the 210s.

90 pounds lost, 5 lb star from WW.

95 pounds lost, 5 lb star from WW.

96.6 pounds lost, weight 209, so in the 200s.

100 pounds, 5 lb star, 100 lbs charm from WW. Get free lifetime membership in WW.

"Glam" photo shoot in tailored suit.

Thank you all for your support!

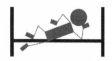

Mixed in among the continuous outpouring of support and love I got from my friends both on Facebook and in the real world were some well-meaning but unconstructive comments, which I took in stride. Others who saw me only two or three times a year were so shocked by my change in appearance that they were concerned I was sick and I raced to reassure them I was fine and that I had done everything under medical supervision. What looked sudden to them seeing the "montage" version was a slow, steady weight-loss over many months.

There were others, however...

There were others who offered comments I can only describe as attempted sabotage.

One friend repeatedly explained to me how losing weight was impossible and keeping it off impossible too (despite the inherent conflict in that statement). One said it was clear my Facebook posts were all lies, and that everyone knew it was all lies and were laughing at me behind my back. Others that said I was trying to commit suicide by starving myself to death and wouldn't taking poison be faster?

Extremely unpleasant, and all from people with serious weight issues of their own in whatever direction. Apparently, I was showing that escape from the Island of Fatness was possible and they found that threatening. As Steven Barnes, *New York Times* bestselling author and martial artist says, "some people don't want to believe that their behavior influences their results."

These were rare cases; most people I shared fatness with cheered me on, which was tremendously helpful. They also asked what I was doing and how I was sticking to it which was also tremendously helpful. Answering their questions made me seriously think about what I was going through and how I was coping and is part of what led me to write this book. Thanks to you all.

Ramblings

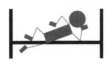

There are lots of things people claim will boost your weight loss in one way or another. Sort of the flip side of the people telling you what not to eat. Some of them do nothing; some of them cost a lot of money and do nothing; some of them can put your health at risk.

Power Foods: There are no "foods you need to eat to lose weight!" as the headlines shout. Some foods have more nutrition than others, some have more calories than others, but that's all there is to it. There's a different right mix of foods for everyone.

Supplements: There is no vitamin, herb or any other such magic-in-a-bottle that will help you lose weight. It's a good idea during any diet to check in with your doctor about what vitamins you might be low on and ask how best to make up the difference (when I started my diet I was very low on vitamins B and D).

Juice Fasts: If you are otherwise healthy there is nothing inherently wrong with juice fasts. You can't do them very long without dying, of course, and any weight you lose during one will come right back when you stop. You'll also pee a lot.

Cleanses: It's the job of your liver and kidneys to clear out all undefined "toxins" in your blood stream on a regular basis and they are doing so as you read this. There is also no need to clear out any part of your body that you empty regularly anyway. If anything was stuck in there, I promise you'd know it.

To Sum Up: fasts, cleanses, supplements, or anything along those lines can be hard on the body. Check with your doctor to make sure you're not putting your health at risk.

How I Dined Out

April 25, 2016

One-Day-Early Tuesday Weight Report:

(I am flying out tomorrow morning and wouldn't have been able to weigh in tomorrow.)

I have lost 2.2 (two-point-two) pounds since last week, putting me at 243 lbs even for a total weight loss of 62.6 pounds over 28 weeks. Since my goal is to reach 205, that leaves me another 37.4 pounds to go. At my current average weight loss of 2.2 pounds per week, that leaves me with another 17.0 weeks to go.

Upcoming Benchmarks:

65 pounds lost, 5 lb star from WW.

66.6 pounds lost, 239 pounds, two-thirds of the way to goal and into the 230s.

70 pounds lost, 5 lb star from WW.

75 pounds lost, three-quarters of the way toward my goal. 5 lb star from WW, 75 lbs lost charm from WW.

76.6 pounds lost, weight at 229, and into the 220s.

80 pounds lost, try on next-size-down pants. 5 lb star from WW.

85 pounds lost, 5 lb star from WW.

85.6 pounds lost, I will be "Overweight" rather than "Obese."

86.6 pounds lost, weight 219, so in the 210s.

90 pounds lost, 5 lb star from WW.

95 pounds lost, 5 lb star from WW.

96.6 pounds lost, weight 209, so in the 200s.

100 pounds, 5 lb star, 100 lbs charm from WW. Get free lifetime membership in WW.

"Glam" photo shoot in tailored suit!

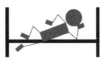

I realized early on that I would have to minimize eating out (and eliminate take-out completely) to stick to my diet. It's hard enough sticking to plan when cooking at home let alone when it's uncertain what is being put in the food. I'm not concerned with whether the burger I'm eating is really beef, or even what part of the cow it's from, but I did wonder how it was being cooked. Did they broil it in butter? It says grilled but do they marinate it in oil first, or pour stuff on it while it's cooking? How many calories are in the teriyaki sauce anyway? It was a bit of a problem, because without being able to join friends for dinner I became even more of a hermit than I already was (I work from home and only visit consulting clients once in a while). How could I ever meet friends at a restaurant? On top of that, how could I be certain that, handed a menu with dozens or even hundreds of tasty items, I would always pick the right thing?

There is this wonderful thing these days called the web. Restaurants put their menus up on it. If I was going to meet friends for dinner I would pick a time during the day when I was not hungry, or rather, less hungry than I might be later, and pick out in advance what I was going to have. That way I didn't even have to open the menu when I got there and avoided the temptation.

Ordering without even opening the menu has the side effect of making someone appear knowledgeable, worldly, and sophisticated (or so I told myself). I limited myself to items that are pretty much the same wherever I went, or would ask them to just leave off anything I couldn't have or replace it with something I could have. Being picky about how exactly my meal is prepared also made me seem knowledgeable, worldly, and sophisticated (I told myself that, too).

None of that prevents an over-eager server who responds to "just coffee for me" at dessert time from hitting you with "Are you sure, we have a wonderful peach pie!" or some such. If a polite "no, thank you" didn't work, I'd switch to a withering stare combined with repeating "No" as many times as it took.

I also worked on making companionship the reason for the gathering rather than merely an accessory to the food. I would ask my friends about their lives and then actually pay attention to their answers, and even ask follow-up questions. Since my friends are, on the whole, fairly entertaining, this approach really worked. It also kept me from treating stuffing my face as the only truly entertaining thing about the gathering.

Traveling on 1500 Calories a Day

May 3, 2016

Tuesday Weight Report:

Despite our week away, I have lost 1.6 lb one-point-six) pounds since last week, putting me at 241.4 lbs for at a total weight loss of 64.2 pounds over 29 weeks. Since my goal is to reach 205, that leaves me another 35.8 pounds to go. At my current average weight loss of 2.2 pounds per week, that leaves me with another 16.3 weeks to go.

Upcoming Benchmarks:

65 pounds lost, 5 lb star from WW.

66.6 pounds lost, 239 pounds, two-thirds of the way to goal and into the 230s.

70 pounds lost, 5 lb star from WW.

75 pounds lost, three-quarters of the way toward my goal. 5 lb star from WW, 75 lbs lost charm from WW.

76.6 pounds lost, weight at 229, and into the 220s.

80 pounds lost, try on next-size-down pants. 5 lb star from WW.

85 pounds lost, 5 lb star from WW.

85.6 pounds lost, I will be "Overweight" rather than "Obese."

86.6 pounds lost, weight 219, so in the 210s.

90 pounds lost, 5 lb star from WW.

95 pounds lost, 5 lb star from WW.

96.6 pounds lost, weight 209, so in the 200s.

100 pounds, 5 lb star, 100 lbs charm from WW. Get free lifetime membership in WW. "Glam" photo shoot in tailored suit.

Thank you all for your support.

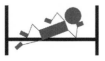

Vacations are really hard on a diet. Travel typically means being out of control of what and when I eat, and that can be a huge problem. A vacation is usually thought of as a time with fewer limitations than in your regular life. For me vacations at hotels with all-you-can-eat breakfasts, well, the breakfast bar was the whole point of staying at a hotel.

While I couldn't eliminate the problem completely, I buckled down and got obsessive. I made sure the hotel we were staying at had in-room cooking facilities. I found a local grocery store that we could shop at or order delivery from on-line. I cut myself some slack and accepted that we would be eating out at least one meal a day, and searched the local restaurants for places that had things that fit into my diet so we could go there.

This research turned up some things I didn't know, like that crab legs, if I didn't pour butter all over them, fit exactly into my diet. Bonus: I found a local restaurant that had a mermaid swimming in a pool in the corner. There are some parts of the human soul that can be fed without food. I also made sure there were plenty of non-food activities that I would find interesting, like being alone in a hotel room with my wife while our son was off surfing for a few hours. Which tops the breakfast bar by a heck of a lot.

Food Pushers and Food Pornographers

May 10, 2016

Tuesday Weight Report:

I have lost 3.0 lbs (three-point-zero) pounds since last week, putting me at 238.4 lbs, for a total weight loss of 67.2 pounds over 30 weeks. Since my goal is to reach 205, that leaves me another 32.8 pounds to go. At my current average weight loss of 2.24 pounds per week, that leaves me with another 14.6 weeks to go.

Benchmarks Achieved:

65 pounds lost, 5 lb star from WW.

66.6 pounds lost, 239 pounds or less, two-thirds of the way to goal and into the 230s.

Upcoming Benchmarks:

70 pounds lost, 5 lb star from WW.

75 pounds lost, three-quarters of the way toward my goal. 5 lb star from WW, 75 lbs lost charm from WW.

76.6 pounds lost, weight at 229, and into the 220s.

80 pounds lost, try on next-size-down pants. 5 lb star from WW.

85 pounds lost, 5 lb star from WW.

85.6 pounds lost, I will be "Overweight" rather than "Obese."

86.6 pounds lost, weight 219, so in the 210s.

90 pounds lost, 5 lb star from WW.

95 pounds lost, 5 lb star from WW.

96.6 pounds lost, weight 209, so in the 200s.

100 pounds, 5 lb star, 100 lbs charm from WW. Get free lifetime membership in WW.

"Glam" photo shoot in tailored suit.

Thank you all for your support!

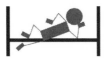

I go visit some friends and they offer me food that is not on my diet one way or another and get upset when I turn down the snack. Often it's because they want a snack but don't want to eat by themselves in front of me, or they want to justify their snacking by my presence, or even that they only invited me over as an excuse to eat. These are the Food Pushers.

In my kinder moments, which are few and far between, I called them Eating Buddies. Drinking buddies you only get together with at a bar and only with the purpose of getting drunk together, whatever else you might tell yourself. As a non-drinker I was surprised to find eating buddies are exactly the same way but with food. It matters a lot to them that I join in the eating. If I said no they'd accept that, but a mutual friend would come up to me and say "it's really hurting his/her feelings that I won't try the < food not on my diet > that she worked on all day" or even "that you not eating < food not on my diet > makes him/her feel fat." I found that if I did break down and have a piece of whatever, they would celebrate my moment of weakness.

I did find in most cases if I called the person before or after and told them how that made things harder for me they would apologize but then simply not invite me to the next gathering because they didn't want to make things hard for me.

There are many reasons losing weight is isolating, but this is a major one.

As for the Food Pornographers, is all but impossible to watch broadcast or basic cable TV without having fried chicken, tacos, or lovingly and unrealistically presented burgers of one kind or another thrust into your face at the size of whatever TV screen is in front of you. In fact I'll go further: it is impossible. The goal of food-chain commercials, whether for fast food or slow food, is to make people hungry. If they can make them want their brand of food right that second, even better.

Millions of dollars and countless hours of psychological and creative effort is focused on that goal. It's behavioral manipulation focused on appetite enhancement. If the same amount of time, effort and money were focused on actual pornography, everyone would be so busy with do-it-yourself orgasms that the human race would be on the edge of dying out.

Not to mention there are entire basic cable channels devoted to ritualized food worship.

Against this sea of advertising I had a mixed, rag-tag fleet of options. I recorded my shows and played them back later, fast-forwarding through the commercials (although there is a whole science devoted to making commercials effective even at high speed), I paid extra for premium channels and subscribed to a number of commercial-free streaming services.

I also read a lot of books. No commercials, no advertisements, and so on, just words in a row. When I ran out of books I wrote one: The one you are reading right now and will buy for all your friends whether they are overweight or not because it makes a great gift for the holidays or any other occasion!

Is Lying There Really Okay?

May 17, 2016
Tuesday Weight Report:
I have lost .6 lbs (point six) pounds since last week, putting me at 237.8 lbs, for a total weight loss of 67.8 pounds over 31 weeks. Since my goal is to reach 205, that leaves me another 32.0 pounds to go. At my current average weight loss of 2.18 pounds per week, that leaves me with another 14.6 weeks to go, same as last week.

Last Friday I did 1 mile on the treadmill over 25 minutes, the last quarter at a 2.5 incline, and came off it absolutely ravenous, which impacted my entire week, reinforcing my construct that my "hunger switch" is broken. I am told that being hungry after exercise is normal, but this was extreme.

I am not giving up on the exercise, but am now forewarned. I've been told by a metabolic specialist to bring 100 calories in low glycemic index carbs with me - like half a cucumber or a handful of raspberries...and eat it immediately after exercising. So I'll give that a shot. The exercise has benefit beyond burning calories and I will concentrate on that.

Upcoming Benchamarks:
70 pounds lost, 5 lb star from WW.
75 pounds lost, three-quarters of the way toward my goal. 5 lb star from WW, 75 lbs lost charm from WW.
76.6 pounds lost, weight at 229, and into the 220s.
80 pounds lost, try on next-size-down pants. 5 lb star from WW.
85 pounds lost, 5 lb star from WW85.6 pounds lost, I will be "Overweight" rather than "Obese."
86.6 pounds lost, weight 219, so in the 210s.
90 pounds lost, 5 lb star from WW.
95 pounds lost, 5 lb star from WW.
96.6 pounds lost, weight 209, so in the 200s.

100 pounds, 5 lb star, 100 lbs charm from WW. Get free lifetime membership in WW.

"Glam" photo shoot in tailored suit.

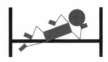

Despite what I said above I did give up on the exercise. It's not that exercise is a bad thing. For me exercise was simply not compatible with losing weight. Nor was it necessary. I was losing weight steadily despite a lack of exercise; that was a reality that was surprising but obvious from the numbers I was racking up. Reality has to intrude sometime.

So I was losing weight, but without exercise was I really getting healthier? Yes, I was. Over the course of my diet I went from having serious GERD, also known as acid reflux, to not having reflux at all. I went from having sleep apnea, which wakes a sufferer up a hundred or more times a night without realizing it because their airway is blocked, to not having sleep apnea. Apnea, by the way, does more than just disrupt sleep, it can be deadly and the exhaustion it causes can, annoyingly, lead to weight gain, which makes the apnea worse, and so on. I stopped snoring, which my wife greatly appreciated.

I was able to get off my cholesterol medication, not because I was eating so little cholesterol, but because fat on the body generates cholesterol. Getting rid of the fat brought my so-called "bad" cholesterol way down and my so-called "good" cholesterol remained the same. My blood pressure however remained too high. So did my tachycardia, both my general too-rapid heart rate and my occasional palpitations (a very too-rapid heart rate). Being overweight is not the only reason for high blood pressure or rapid heart rates by a long shot. Fat people very often get lousy healthcare. More to come on that.

Fat People Get Lousy Healthcare

May 24, 2016

Tuesday Weight Report:

I have lost 3.6 lbs (three point six) pounds since last week, putting me at 234.2 lbs, for a total weight loss of 71.4 pounds over 32 weeks. Since my goal is to reach 205, that leaves me another 28.6 pounds to go. At my current average weight loss of 2.23 pounds per week, that leaves me with another 12.8 weeks to go.

It could be that last week I got a little slippery on my program and so only lost .6, it could be nothing more than the expected unevenness of weight-loss. What matters most is maintaining the average weight loss of just over 2 pounds a week.

Thank you all for your support!

Benchmarks Achieved:

70 pounds lost, 5 lb star from WW.

Upcoming Benchmarks:

75 pounds lost, three-quarters of the way toward my goal. 5 lb star from WW, 75 lbs lost charm from WW.

76.6 pounds lost, weight at 229, and into the 220s.

80 pounds lost, try on next-size-down pants. 5 lb star from WW.

85 pounds lost, 5 lb star from WW.

85.6 pounds lost, I will be "Overweight" rather than "Obese."

86.6 pounds lost, weight 219, so in the 210s.

90 pounds lost, 5 lb star from WW.

95 pounds lost, 5 lb star from WW.

96.6 pounds lost, weight 209, so in the 200s.

100 pounds, 5 lb star, 100 lbs charm from WW. Get free lifetime membership in WW.

"Glam" photo shoot in tailored suit.

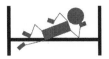

Doctors do not always suck. I owe my life and current slim figure in great part to doctors. As with all professions, though, some doctors do suck. Some are good at one thing but not at another. Maybe it was just my bad luck that I had so many doctors that assumed all my health issues were related to my weight, and told me to go lose weight to get rid of them, as if that were easy. It was like being told "the cure for all your health problems is on top of Mount Everest; just climb on up there and grab it." It was something that seems doable, because there are a hundred people so a year who do climb Everest, but not practical advice for 99.9 percent of the patients a doctor sees. My doctors before Dr. Case did not treat my high blood pressure or too-rapid heart rate, they just told me those things would go away if I lost weight.

When I saw Dr. Case I was over 300 pounds, 309 on his scale. After examination and testing, he immediately put me on meds for high cholesterol, high blood pressure and rapid heart rate. Only then did we discuss losing weight. I was floored to find a doctor who treated what was wrong with me as I presented and whose attitude was more "the only way to figure out which of these symptoms are caused by you being overweight is for you to lose weight." He then accepted that as a fat person, I knew how to lose weight, the challenge was, as always, keeping it off. He basically ordered me to get the weight off first and then we'd work on how to keep it off. Then he kept faith with me when I fell off the wagon and had to start over.

As it turns out my high blood pressure and rapid heartbeat are due to a minor genetic condition that has nothing to do with my weight, something I might never have known if Dr. Case hadn't started me on the meds first thing.

I'd Rather Lose Weight

May 31, 2016

Tuesday Weight Report:

I have lost 1.8 lbs (one-point-eight) pounds since last week, putting me at 232.4 lbs, for a total weight loss of 73.2 pounds over 33 weeks. Since my goal is to reach 205, that leaves me another 26.8 pounds to go. At my current average weight loss of 2.21 pounds per week, that leaves me with another 12.1 weeks to go.

Technically this week's loss was slightly below the average I want to maintain of 2 lbs a week, but I had to seriously rehydrate this week; a low-sodium diet carries a risk of dehydration and I had fallen into that trap. So I'm happy with the outcome.

Thank you all for your support!

Upcoming Benchmarks:

75 pounds lost, three-quarters of the way toward my goal. 5 lb star from WW, 75 lbs lost charm from WW.

76.6 pounds lost, weight at 229, and into the 220s.

80 pounds lost, try on next-size-down pants. 5 lb star from WW.

85 pounds lost, 5 lb star from WW.

85.6 pounds lost, I will be "Overweight" rather than "Obese."

86.6 pounds lost, weight 219, so in the 210s.

90 pounds lost, 5 lb star from WW.

95 pounds lost, 5 lb star from WW.

96.6 pounds lost, weight 209, so in the 200s.

100 pounds, 5 lb star, 100 lbs charm from WW. Get free lifetime membership in WW.

"Glam" photo shoot in tailored suit.

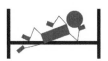

One of my biggest battles was fighting the urge to have "just one more helping" or increase my portion by just a little. Or skip the bother of measuring out a portion and just eyeball the amount (that trick never works). Or snag a snack I happened to be walking by, or give in to any of the thousand temptations a day that happen in a culture where food basically falls from the sky on a regular basis. It really was, and is, a constant mental battle.

So what I did in those situations was focus on how good it felt to weigh in at the end of a week having lost weight. Remembering that feeling was usually enough to get me to keep my hand at my side instead of reaching for what was unexpectedly on offer. Another option was simply leaving the situation; if I had to I would cross the street to avoid walking past a group of food trucks and food carts or windows-open-to-the-street pizza vendors. Easier said than done, but it was all part of killing my food-to-mouth reflex. Also, as I discussed in the Just Rewards section, it helped to treat myself to something that wasn't food.

Feed a Cold, Feed a Fever

June 7, 2016
Tuesday Weight Report:
I have lost 1.2 lbs (one-point-two pounds) since last week, putting me at 231.2 lbs for a total weight loss of 74.4 pounds over 34 weeks. Since my goal is to reach 205, that leaves me another 25.6 pounds to go. At my current average weight loss of 2.18 pounds per week, that leaves me with another 11.7 weeks to go.

This week's loss is certainly below the average I am trying to maintain of 2 lbs a week, but I am still fighting dehydration and I've been told by a metabolic specialist that at this point in my program a target of 1.5 lbs a week is more rational. Still, I'm going to cut my portion size by 1/5th and see what happens this next week.

And yes, it's annoying to be this close to a nice round 75 lbs lost, but I refuse to be upset that I "only" lost 1.2 lbs this week, and if I do the same next week, that's fine too.

Thank you all for your support!

Upcoming Benchmarks:
75 pounds lost, three-quarters of the way toward my goal. 5 lb star from WW, 75 lbs lost charm from WW.
76.6 pounds lost, weight at 229, and into the 220s.
80 pounds lost, try on next-size-down pants. 5 lb star from WW
85 pounds lost, 5 lb star from WW.
85.6 pounds lost, I will be "Overweight" rather than "Obese."
86.6 pounds lost, weight 219, so in the 210s.
90 pounds lost, 5 lb star from WW.
95 pounds lost, 5 lb star from WW.
96.6 pounds lost, weight 209, so in the 200s.

100 pounds, 5 lb star, 100 lbs charm from WW. Get free lifetime membership in WW.

"Glam" photo shoot in tailored suit.

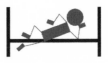

When I'm sick, I want to eat. Call it my approach to alternative medicine. If I have a nasty headache, I apply pizza. If I'm running a fever, I apply bacon cheeseburgers. If my stomach is upset, I apply Chinese food, if I throw it up, I apply more Chinese food because that empty stomach makes me even hungrier. Sunburn? Chocolate Milkshake. Heartburn? Vanilla Milkshake. Burn my tongue? Tacos. Well, soft tacos. The reflex to eat when I'm stressed is ten times stronger when I'm not feeling well.

I coped using two methods: When I was sick I slept as much as I could, and I complained, well, whined, a lot to my wife. "I feel like crap and I want to eat all the pastrami!" I would shout. "Yes, Dear," she would say. "Poor John!" Did she mean that sincerely? I have no idea. I don't look a possibly sympathetic wife in the mouth. I just asked her to bring me Motrin or Pepto or Imodium or whatever else I needed, and tried to groan out a weak thanks. And oh yes. For diarrhea? Fried mozzarella sticks. What else?

Unlisted Benchmarks

June 14, 2016

Tuesday Weight Report:

I have lost 1.6 lbs (one-point-six pounds) since last week, putting me at 229.6 lbs for a total weight loss of 76.0 pounds over 35 weeks. Since my goal is to reach 205, that leaves me another 24.6 pounds to go. At my current average weight loss of 2.17 pounds per week, that leaves me with another 11 weeks to go.

However, despite my dropping my portions/calories by 1/5th, it appears my metabolic specialist was correct: having lost 25% of my body weight, my caloric need has dropped to the point where a reasonable loss per week expectation is more like 1.5 than 2.0.

Thank you all for your support!

Benchmarks Achieved:

76 pounds lost, over three-quarters of the way toward my goal. 5 lb star from WW, 75 lbs lost charm from WW.

76 pounds lost, into the 220s.

Benchmarks to Come:

80 pounds lost, try on next-size-down pants. 5 lb star from WW.

85 pounds lost, 5 lb star from WW.

85.6 pounds lost, I will be "Overweight" rather than "Obese."

86 pounds lost, weight 219 lbs, so in the 210s.

90 pounds lost, 5 lb star from WW.

95 pounds lost, 5 lb star from WW.

96 pounds lost, weight 209 lbs so in the 200s.

100 pounds, 5 lb star, 100 lbs charm from WW. Get free lifetime membership in WW.

"Glam" photo shoot in tailored suit.

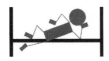

I've been listing the benchmarks I set for myself, but once in a while I would notice something I hadn't thought of in advance that was kind of the Universe telling me I'd passed one of *its* benchmarks.

<u>On April 19th, 2016</u>, my wedding ring slipped off my finger. This meant I was thinner than I had been at my wedding 17 years earlier. On the same day I fit into a bathing suit purchased in desperation at a hotel a year earlier.

<u>On April 26th, 2016</u>, I discovered I no longer needed a seat belt extender on airplanes.

<u>On April 28th, 2016</u>, I got the blood tests back from my annual physical. I was no longer even slightly pre-diabetic. There was nothing that even hinted at diabetes any more.

<u>On May 12th, 2016</u>, I noticed that getting up and getting things was easier than I could remember it being, and that going into another room and finding stuff myself annoyed people a lot less than lying there and shouting for them to fetch me things. Who'd have thought?

<u>On July 5th, 2016</u>, I realized I could now reach anywhere on my back that itched and was no longer dependent on friends and family to do it for me.

<u>On September 10th, 2016</u>, I hit waist size 40, which meant I had dropped out of the Big and Tall shops and was now in the upper range for regular men's department.

Holiday Meals

June 21, 2016
Tuesday Weight Report:
I have lost 2.6 lbs (two-point-six pounds) since last week, putting me at 227.0 lbs for a total weight loss of 78.6 pounds over 36 weeks. Since my goal is to reach 205, that leaves me another 22.0 pounds to go. At my current average weight loss of 2.18 pounds per week, that leaves me with another 10 weeks to go.

Apparently switching from grains to greens put me back on track.
Thank you all for your support!
Benchmarks to Come:
80 pounds lost, try on next-size-down pants. 5 lb star from WW.
85 pounds lost, 5 lb star from WW.
85.6 pounds lost, I will be "Overweight" rather than "Obese."
86 pounds lost, weight 219 lbs so in the 210s.
90 pounds lost, 5 lb star from WW.
95 pounds lost, 5 lb star from WW.
96 pounds lost, weight 209 lbs so in the 200s.
100 pounds, 5 lb star, 100 lbs charm from WW. Get free lifetime membership in WW.
"Glam" photo shoot in tailored suit.

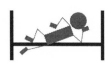

I made it through meals with family on the holidays by hosting them myself. I found that if I were in control of every part of the meal, not only what I was making myself but what everyone else was going to bring, I could make certain that there were things on the menu that I could enjoy. That I wouldn't be walking into a Temptation Alley where I would be faced with a huge spread of things, none of which I could eat. Yes, it meant getting stuck with the cooking and the cleaning up after (although we could count on our friends and relatives swooping down on the dishes like vultures on a rotting corpse, or perhaps a less grotesque simile) but hey, the host is always the one who never has time to eat anything because they are so busy looking after things.

And don't think we had to skimp on the delicacies! Being in charge of the menu meant that I could make versions of things that were accessible to me that everyone would love, and have them bring things that others would love (and some things I could have as well). Or provide things I don't happen to enjoy like cranberry sauce or sweet potatoes. Didn't matter what was in them if I didn't want to eat them, and more for everyone else. So as with every other part of this diet, holiday meals were a matter of balance and control.

Want is Not Wrong

June 28, 2016
Tuesday Weight Report:
I have lost 1.6 lbs (one-point-six pounds) since last week, putting me at 225.4 lbs, for a total weight loss of 80.2 pounds over 37 weeks. Since my goal is to reach 205, that leaves me another 20.4 pounds to go. At my current average weight loss of 2.16 pounds per week, that leaves me with another 9.5 weeks to go.
Benchmarks Achieved:
80 pounds lost, try on next-size-down pants. 5 lb star from WW.
Thank you all for your support!
Benchmarks to Come:
85 pounds lost, 5 lb star from WW.
85.6 pounds lost, I will be "Overweight" rather than "Obese."
86 pounds lost, weight 219.?, so in the 210s.
90 pounds lost, 5 lb star from WW.
95 pounds lost, 5 lb star from WW.
96 pounds lost, weight 209 lbs so in the 200s.
100 pounds, 5 lb star, 100 lbs charm from WW. Get free lifetime membership in WW.
"Glam" photo shoot in tailored suit.

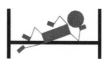

I want food every time I see it. Doesn't matter if it's a steak or a cake or freaking Jell-O, I want to eat it. It is extremely annoying. Even if I just ate, looking at food makes me hunger for it.

I used to think that made me a bad person, that it meant something was morally wrong with me, that I was a glutton, and gluttony is of course one of the Seven Deadly Sins of the Flesh. Fat people are treated like slothful sinners anyway, so that's two of the Deadlies right there. Being fat was my own fault due to my own sin.

Nothing could be further from the truth.

There is a Christian concept of "adultery in the heart" which means that being tempted to commit a sin is as bad as committing it. That concept is so much a part of our culture that even I, a Jewish kid from New York, somehow picked it up. I no longer think that in any way. Being tempted by something that I know I should resist is a burden to carry, not a sin. I would much rather not react so strongly to food but I no longer feel bad about it when I do. It's just a fact of my life that I have to watch out for if I want to stay thin.

Sex Stuff

July 5, 2016

Tuesday Weight Report:

I have lost .4 lbs (point-four pounds) since last week, putting me at 225 lbs for a total weight loss of 80.6 pounds over 38 weeks. Since my goal is to reach 205, that leaves me another 20 pounds to go. At my current average weight loss of 2.12 pounds per week, that leaves me with another 9.43 weeks to go.

Would have liked to lose more weight this week; I attribute the slower weight loss to being a bit sloppy with my eating management and to having eaten a LOT of MSG this past week...yes, I mean more than a few spoonfuls. Some people supposedly get headaches from the stuff, I get a buzz. So I'm off MSG now.

Thank you all for your support!

Benchmarks to Come:

85 pounds lost, 5 lb star from WW.

85.6 pounds lost, I will be "Overweight" rather than "Obese."

86 pounds lost, weight 219.?, so in the 210s.

90 pounds lost, 5 lb star from WW.

95 pounds lost, 5 lb star from WW.

96 pounds lost, weight 209 lbs so in the 200s.

100 pounds, 5 lb star, 100 lbs charm from WW. Get free lifetime membership in WW.

"Glam" photo shoot in tailored suit.

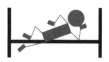

I really like sex, which I don't think makes me all that different from most people reading this. How often, with whom, and how many people are involved in a given week, month, year, or bed is none of anyone's business. I won't be going into any detail about my sex life with my beautiful wife except to say that whether I was fat or thin or in between my wife and I got along just fine in that area.

However, I find sex to be much more frequent and much more – flexible – now that I am thinner. I'm simply up for it more often, can maneuver more easily, last longer (in the without-feeling-faint sense, not the other sense) and am basically more likely to choose sex over sleep than I was. My reaction to being asked "Honey, would you like to go to the bedroom?" is no longer "sex would be great but I'd have to get to my feet and climb up all those stairs and I'll be so tired that it won't amount to much anyway so I might as well stay here," but "Sure!" Sex is good and good for you, and it is my favorite of the "non-food rewards" I mentioned earlier. I recommend it.

Ramblings

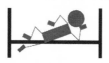

There are things about metabolism that the word-on-the-street gets consistently wrong. For example:

Set-point: there is no such thing as a "set point," a certain weight your body will maintain in some automatic way and that can somehow be reset. Everyone eats when they are hungry and stops when they are full, then starts eating again when they're hungry again. It's as simple and annoying as that. What's different between naturally thin people and fat people is that naturally thin people fill up faster and don't get hungry as often. Some people will eat two cookies and put the rest of the bag back because they are satisfied. Others will just keep eating until the bag is empty (I am in that latter group). If there is some way to convert one kind of person into the other, no one has come up with it.

Speeding up metabolism: other than using incredibly dangerous drugs there is no way to speed up metabolism so calories burn off at a significantly higher rate. Exercise will burn calories, but it won't change metabolic rate and as in my case can increase hunger. I first heard this phrase from Karla Fisher, a former personal trainer I met on Facebook: "Weight is lost in the kitchen, not in the gym." There is simply no way to take your eyes off the ball and eat by reflex. Boy I wish there were.

Muscle burns calories faster than fat: this one is somewhat true, but that doesn't mean fat cells burn zero calories and muscles burn a whole lot. Overall someone will lose six more calories an hour if they are well-muscled than if they aren't. They'll also quite likely be hungrier. That's the reason why a 300 pound linebacker and a 300 pound fat person eat about the same amount (during off season at least).

Fat Can't Change Into Muscle: fat is fuel, it can only be burned. Muscles can be grown and made bigger, stronger and more limber. There is no alchemy that can change one into the other.

Stomachs do not shrink: While you can certainly reduce your waistline, the digestive organ inside you stays the same size throughout your life. You can accustom yourself to smaller meals, but the size of your stomach never changes.

You can't target fat: You can chose a part of the body to build muscle on or firm the muscle in, but your body puts on and loses weight in a set manner that differs between men and women.

Starvation Mode: this is the idea that when someone diets for a while their body adjusts to the lower food intake in such a way that they stop losing weight. Clearly if this were true no one would ever starve. What's really going on is that when their body mass drops, their caloric need drops, so to continue losing weight they have to cut calories even further. Which means smaller portions. Which is a pain.

When it comes to weight loss another phrase passed on by Karla Fisher sums it up for me: "embrace the suck."

Losing Weight for Yourself and Others

July 12, 2016
Tuesday Weight Report:
I have lost 3.4 lbs (three-point-four pounds) since last week, putting me at 221.6 lbs, for a total weight loss of 84 pounds over 39 weeks. Since my goal is to reach 205, that leaves me another 16 pounds to go. At my current average weight loss of 2.15 pounds per week, that leaves me with another 7.4 weeks to go.

I think a combination of no MSG and sticking strictly to my program really helped.

No Benchmarks this week but I do now have less than 20 lbs to go, and there are several Benchmarks I hope to hit in the next couple of weeks. :)

Thank you all for your support!
Benchmarks to Come:
85 pounds lost, 5 lb star from WW.
85.6 pounds lost, I will be "Overweight" rather than "Obese."
86 pounds lost, weight 219.?, so in the 210s.
90 pounds lost, 5 lb star from WW.
95 pounds lost, 5 lb star from WW.
96 pounds lost, weight 209 lbs so in the 200s.
100 pounds, 5 lb star, 100 lbs charm from WW. Get free lifetime membership in WW.

"Glam" photo shoot in tailored suit.

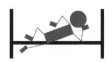

Recurring advice I was given along the way was that if my life was all filled up with taking care of others, I should learn it was also important to take care of myself for myself. That I was important too, etc. I don't quite agree with that, because that way of thinking makes two competing needs out of what is really just one. Someone who takes care of themselves is in a better shape to take care of others and will be around for them that much longer.

In my case, my son is autistic and will likely need a high level of support the rest of his life. That means he is going to need his parents around as long as we can manage to be here. Plus my wife says she needs me around as long as possible too. Getting my health in order to maximize my time on Earth is taking care of them as well as taking care of myself. I know it is a blessing for me and my family that my mother, in her late 80s, is still up and running (with a new hip) and able to be a big help in our lives. The least I can do is try to be there for my wife and son the same way. That it also happens to make me both look and feel better is a huge plus. It's a win-win.

How People See Me

July 19, 2106
Tuesday Weight Report:
I have lost .6 lbs (point six pounds) since last week, putting me at 221.0 lbs, for a total weight loss of 84.6 pounds over 40 weeks. Since my goal is to reach 205.6 that leaves me another 15.4 pounds to go. At my current average weight loss of 2.11 pounds per week, that leaves me with another 7.29 weeks to go.

(For those who saw the earlier version of this post: I decided that a goal of 100 lbs lost is enough, and have moved the number I'm trying to reach to 205.6. When I get there we'll see what I have to do next.))

I attribute the lower-than-average weight-loss to various factors: being sloppy in my diet, significant lost sleep, and my trying a somewhat different approach to eating. This next week will see a return to my usual approach. I'm trying out some different approaches as I see the end of the diet looming and will have to transition to a less restrictive program.

No Benchmarks this week but I did get the pants I was owed, and I am down from size 52 pants to size 42 pants. Oh, and I get to be obese at least one more week! :)

Thank you all for your support!
Benchmarks to Come:
85 pounds lost, 5 lb star from WW.
85.6 pounds lost, I will be "Overweight" rather than "Obese."
86 pounds lost, weight 219.?, so in the 210s.
90 pounds lost, 5 lb star from WW.
95 pounds lost, 5 lb star from WW.
96 pounds lost, weight 209 lbs so in the 200s.
100 pounds, 5 lb star, 100 lbs charm from WW. Get free lifetime membership in WW.
"Glam" photo shoot in tailored suit.

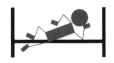

When I was fat I was perceived as unhealthy, unprofessional, and unattractive. Was that fair? No. Was it the reality? Yes. Lots of things about our society are unfair. Although I was unhealthy, most fat people are just fine, thank you, and some thin people are at death's door. Was I unprofessional? I'm sure I could be at times like anyone else. Was I unattractive? My wife denies that, and who am I to doubt her word?

That said, once I'd lost the weight, and was able to dress well, how people saw me changed completely. I was now, if I say so myself, dapper, in large part because I was now able to dress well but also because I was comfortable in nice clothing. It seemed worth it to buy and wear nice clothing because when I was fat I always felt like no matter how I gussied up I'd just be thought of as a fat guy. Whether I was right about that or not, that's how I felt.

Once I'd dropped the weight and was looking and feeling good people were reacting to me on a completely different level. Women were chatting me up. One said to me at a party "Have we met? I feel like I know you from somewhere" which is a very old line but no one had used a line on me in decades. People I had never met saw me as professional and competent and listened with noticeably greater attention to what I had to say and my input on a problem (people who knew me had already formed their own opinions). Do I enjoy that new perception? Yes. But it also bothers me a bit that all I had changed was my weight and what I wore, nothing about myself.

Celebrating the Day I Became "Overweight."

July 26, 2016
Tuesday Weight Report:
I have lost 2.8 lbs (two-point-eight pounds) since last week, putting me at 218.2 lbs, for a total weight loss of 87.4 pounds over 41 weeks. Since my goal is to reach 205.6 that leaves me another 12.8 pounds to go. At my current average weight loss of 2.13 pounds per week, that leaves me with another 6.1 weeks to go.

Benchmarks Achieved:
Greater than 85 pounds lost, 5 lb star from WW.
Greater than 85.6 pounds lost, I will be "Overweight" rather than "Obese."
87.4 pounds lost, weight 218.2, so in the 210s.
Benchmarks to Come:
90 pounds lost, 5 lb star from WW.
95 pounds lost, 5 lb star from WW.
96 pounds lost, weight 209 lbs so in the 200s.
100 pounds, 5 lb star, 100 lbs charm from WW. Get free lifetime membership in WW.
"Glam" photo shoot in tailored suit.

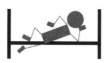

For decades the standard for how much someone should weigh for a given height was computed by the Body Mass Index, or BMI. Those charts show for any given height (I am just under 6'), a range of "normal" weights, and over that range by a certain large amount, the label changes to "obese" which means "really, really fat." Somewhat less over the range you are merely "overweight." I found it highly amusing that I had had to lose 87.4 pounds just to become overweight.

Nowadays the best doctors use a different system, based on height/waist ratio. This system is far more accurate because the BMI does not take into account how much of your body mass comes from muscle rather than fat. The height/waist system does account for that, because as I understand it no matter how much muscle on the body your waist size will stay about the same. Something like that. Any good Primary Care Doctor will be able to explain how the system works.

The Fat Jokers

August 2, 2016
Tuesday Weight Report:
I have lost 1.8 lbs (one-point-eight pounds) since last week, putting me at 216.4 lbs for a total weight loss of 89.2 pounds over 42 weeks. Since my goal is to reach 205.6, that leaves me another 10.8 pounds to go. At my current average weight loss of 2.12 pounds per week, that leaves me with another 5.1 weeks to go.

No benchmarks reached this week, but much self-congratulations because I have a bad cold and really wanted to eat to feel better. :/
Benchmarks to Come:
90 pounds lost, 5 lb star from WW.
90+ pounds lost, pounds to go in single digits.
95 pounds lost, 5 lb star from WW.
96 pounds lost, weight 209 lbs so in the 200s.
100 pounds, 5 lb star, 100 lbs charm from WW.
"Glam" photo shoot in tailored suit.

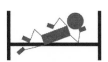

To comedians fat people have a target on their back. Apparently, that's okay because the serious health issue a fat person faces is visible, while someone with the nasal passages of a howler monkey from cocaine or a liver that glows in the dark from booze isn't a target because they still look great in a tight outfit.

Oh, wait, that doesn't make it okay.

That you're not fat doesn't make you smarter or better; it just makes you a bit luckier. Defending trashing people by saying you're encouraging them to lose weight is total bullshit. What you're doing is kicking someone when they are down. You don't get to be cruel to someone, or humiliate or embarrass them because they somehow don't live up to your standards.

Telling you to cut out the fat jokes is not some kind of PC thing, and I'm telling you: cut them out. Fat jokes are too easy, too old, and are punching down.

Comedy is a fantastic medium. Speaking truth to power is vital. Keep it up. It helps keep us sane in these wacky, wacky times. Pointing at the fat kid and laughing helps no one and drops you from insightful observer of the foibles of humanity into the general asshole septic tank.

Man Boobs Away!

August 9, 2016

Tuesday Weight Report:
I have lost 2.2 lbs (two-point-two pounds) since last week, putting me at 214.2 lbs, for a total weight loss of 91.4 pounds over 43 weeks. Since my goal is to reach 205.6 that leaves me another 8.6 pounds to go. At my current average weight loss of 2.12 pounds per week, that leaves me with another 4.05 weeks to go.

Benchmarks Achieved:
90 pounds lost, 5 lb star from WW.
90+ pounds lost, pounds to go in single digits.
Benchmarks to Come:
95 pounds lost, 5 lb star from WW.
96 pounds lost, weight 209 lbs so in the 200s.
100 pounds, 5 lb star, 100 lbs charm from WW.
"Glam" photo shoot in tailored suit.

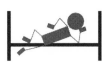

As with many fat men I had very noticeable "man-boobs." Perhaps not ones a Playboy model would envy but enough for me to feel ashamed and, well, unmanly, when I accidentally caught sight of myself in a mirror (I would never look at myself intentionally, clothed or unclothed). I didn't make a note on Facebook when they disappeared, exactly, as I wasn't checking my reflection but eventually I looked down and there they weren't. I had achieved a flat, hairy, unmistakably male chest.

A little to the South, on the other hand, my, uh, manhood grew to three or four times its original impressive size. Or maybe it only seemed that way because my stomach had shrunk to the point where, looking down past my now-manly chest, I could see myself without a mirror.

I'm going to go with my penis grew. Spread the word. It will sell copies of this book.

Visits with Old Friends

August 16, 2016
Tuesday Weight Report:
Neither lost nor gained this week, first time that has happened to me (probably in my life). I had gotten sloppy on portion control, so will have to bear down for this last stretch.

I have lost 0.0 lbs (zero-point-zero pounds) since last week, putting me at 214.2 lbs for a total weight loss of 91.4 pounds over 44 weeks. Since my goal is to reach 205.6 that leaves me another 8.6 pounds to go. At my current average weight loss of 2.07 pounds per week, that leaves me with another 4.15 weeks to go.

Benchmarks to Come:
95 pounds lost, 5 lb star from WW.
96 pounds lost, weight 209 lbs so in the 200s.
100 pounds, 5 lb star, 100 lbs charm from WW.
"Glam" photo shoot in tailored suit.

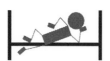

Once I'd lost the weight I took great pleasure in looking up old friends who had not seen me since I shrank. Their reactions, from amazement to completely failing to recognize me, were (and are) a great reward for all the effort I put into losing the weight. If that seems childish and boastful, and me being a show-off, well, yeah, I am those things and I was showing off. Part of it, though, is to keep me on track with my weight. Now that they've seen me thin, now that their image of me has been remade, it keeps me wanting to stay consistent with that image. Heck, I have whole social groups that haven't seen me except in Facebook photos yet. That helps keep me on track too.

Food Dreaming on such a Hungry Day

August 23, 2016
Tuesday Weight Report:
I have lost 4.4 lbs (four-point-four pounds) since last week, putting me at 209.8 lbs for a total weight loss of 95.8 pounds over 45 weeks. Since my goal is to reach 205.6 that leaves me another 4.2 pounds to go. At my current average weight loss of 2.12 pounds per week, that leaves me with another 1.9 weeks to go.
Benchmarks Achieved:
95 pounds lost, 5 lb star from WW.
95.8 pounds lost, weight 209.8 so in the 200s.
Benchmarks to Come:
100 pounds, 5 lb star, 100 lbs charm from WW.
"Glam" photo shoot in tailored suit.

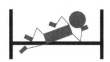

One of the few food-related bright spots along the way was the wonderful nights I would dream of food. Of a lot of food, like the world's largest and most sumptuously laid-out buffet. This came in two variants. In one I would feel horrible for breaking my diet and going to town on the delicious delectables laid out for me, then wake up relived that I hadn't really said to hell with it and thrown all my hard work out the window. The other was the kind of lucid-but-asleep state where you realize you are dreaming and you realize you can eat as much as you want without the slightest qualm. That was my favorite kind, because it was totally guilt-free eating without consequence. I can't speak for everyone who has ever been on a diet, but eating until you are fully and completely satisfied without consequence is literally the dream.

Adopting the Vanity Lifestyle

August 30, 2016
Tuesday Weight Report:
I have lost 3.2 lbs (three-point-two pounds) since last week, putting me at 206.6 lbs for a total weight loss of 99.0 pounds over 46 weeks. Since my goal is to reach 205.6 that leaves me another 1.0 pounds to go. At my current average weight loss of 2.15 pounds per week, that leaves me with another .5 (point five) weeks to go.

I have an appointment with the doctor on Friday at 2 pm to discuss where I stand and whether I should continue to lose weight past the 100 lbs goal I set (more because it was a big round number than for any medical reason) 46 weeks ago.

For those who have expressed concern: I will follow my doctor's guidance. If he says to lose more, I will; if he says not to, I will work on figuring out how to keep weight off, and begin focusing on fitness either way.

Also once I hit 100 lbs down I will most certainly follow through with the benchmark below, so get your equipment ready ! :)
Benchmarks to Come:
100 pounds, 5 lb star, 100 lbs charm from WW.
"Glam" photo shoot in tailored suit.

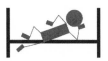

I assume I have the usual assortment of personality flaws, because people tell me I do, even though I don't see them. Among them, I'm told, I can be arrogant and pretentious and a bit of a know-it-all, but if I were, I'd know it, wouldn't I?

That said, the one thing I have never been, up until now, is vain about my appearance. I simply assumed I was a fatty and therefore grotesque and there was nothing I could really do about how I looked. I could dress up in a nice suit and people would say "Hey, look, there's a fat guy in a nice suit!" Since I couldn't win, why even try?

Now that I've lost the weight, though, I find myself spending more and more time at the mirror checking out how I look. I am clean-shaven now instead of sporting the unkempt, badly trimmed beard thing (not that I didn't rock it). I keep my hair nicely styled, I've started using a variety of hair-and-skin products that make me all shiny and new. I'm testing different colognes by putting them on and asking my wife to sniff me. So far she seems to like the chocolate and peppermint ones best, while I prefer the bacon scent (yes, there is bacon scented cologne) which just shows my natural attraction to food. I'm probably going to wind up somewhere between sandalwood and musk.

So now I can add what I hope is a reasonable level of vanity to my other fine qualities.

A Step Back

September 6, 2016
Tuesday Weight Report:
And in the building the suspense department...
I have gained (GAINED) 1.6 (one-point-six pounds) since last week, putting me at 208.2 lbs, for a total weight loss of 97.4 pounds over 48 weeks. Since my goal is to reach 205.6 that leaves me another 2.6 pounds to go. At my current average weight loss of 2.02 pounds per week, that leaves me with another 1.2 weeks to go.

The weight gain is most likely due to my having been dehydrated the last two weeks and having set out to hydrate my ass off. :) Also I probably wasn't as careful as I usually am about portions.
So, onward, head-unbowed! :)
Benchmarks to Come:
100 pounds, 5 lb star, 100 lbs charm from WW.
"Glam" photo shoot in tailored suit.

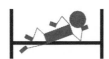

So yeah, while my progress was steady as I went along, I did have some reversals. And yes I did panic. All this effort will have been for naught, as everyone who told me I'd just gain it back turned out to be right and I'm going to put all the weight back on and etc. etc. That was when I leaned on friends and family for support. Once I calmed down, I realized what I had to do: cut my calories by twenty percent yet again. That was not easy to face, but I did it.

No, I wasn't eating three grains of rice with a tweezers and calling it a meal. The portions I ate in this last push were still perfectly reasonable, healthy amounts of food. It was where I was before I started, eating as much as I wanted, which was basically as much as there was around, that made these portions seem like a thimbleful of gruel.

Never Too Old

September 13, 2016

Tuesday Weight Report:

I have lost 1.4 lbs (one-point-four pounds) since last week, putting me at 206.8 lbs, for a total weight loss of 98.8 pounds over 49 weeks. Since my goal is to reach 205.6 that leaves me another 1.2 pounds to go. At my current average weight loss of 2.01 pounds per week, that leaves me with another 0.59 weeks to go.

I have worked extremely hard to keep hydrated this past week, so I feel that this week the weight loss is real, in the sense that it is fat, not water.

I am down to LT size shirts (large/tall) and down to "large" on shorts and in dress pants, from 52 in stretch-waist (which essentially adds another 1.25 possible inches to your waist) where I started, I am now in size 40 classic fit (non-stretch) pants; I have left the big-and-tall store behind at least for now, and hopefully for good.

So tune in next week for the continuing adventure. Is the suspense getting to you? Because it's killing me! :)

Benchmarks to Come:

100 pounds, 5 lb star, 100 lbs charm from WW. "Glam" photo shoot in tailored suit.

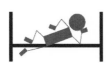

I started my diet when I was 53 years old. I have bounced up and down in weight my whole life and the common wisdom I kept getting was that the older I was, the harder it is to lose weight. I did not find that to be true. I found that the experience of age and knowledge of myself that came with it more than compensated for any reduction there might have in my metabolism.

I found that with age came a certain calmness, patience, and stability that I was sorely lacking in my youth, and a greater ability to focus. Whether that was inevitable or the result of lots of therapy or that I was just generally more secure in my ability to cope with the random crap life throws at me I have no idea.

I wouldn't accept that I had lived as a fat man so long that I had to accept I would die a fat man. There are many things about my life that I cannot change; my weight is no longer one of them.

So Close I Could Taste It

September 20, 2016
Tuesday Weight Report:
I have lost .4 lbs (point-four pounds) since last week, putting me at 206.4 lbs for a total weight loss of 99.2 pounds over 50 weeks. Since my goal is to reach 205.6 that leaves me another .8 pounds to go. At my current average weight loss of 1.98 pounds per week, that leaves me with another 0.4 weeks to go.

Clearly I have hit another plateau, although the swelling in and around my mouth due to ongoing dental work (as well as the effect of medications) may be part of it. The question now is whether I drop calories another 20 percent to get back up to my typical weight loss or just accept it is likely to take a couple of weeks so to hit the 100 lbs down goal. I think I'll try a combo of both.

My face looks a bit beat-up for victory photos at the moment anyway.
Benchmarks to Come:
100 pounds, 5 lb star, 100 lbs charm from WW.
"Glam" photo shoot in tailored suit.

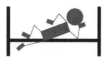

September 21, the day after I posted the above, I posted this:
Confession time. When I started this weight loss thing, I really wanted to drop 100 lbs in a year or less. I am currently 99.2 pounds down and on week 50.

So that let the cat out of the bag. I had not only set a goal of losing one hundred pounds, I had set the goal of doing so within a set period of time. While that is not recommended by any program I know of, it worked for me because it gave a sense of urgency that kept me from slacking off.

I chose to do it in one year because with fifty-two weeks in a year, that meant with an average weight loss of two pounds a week, or even slightly less, I would be able to make the hundred pounds in that length of time.

Per my doctor and many other sources, dropping between one and two pounds a week was safe and healthy and a reasonable thing to expect of myself. If I'd set a goal that was too difficult I would have failed, and too dangerous would have defeated the underlying goal of improving my health.

Rationally I knew it wouldn't make a real difference if I hit my target weight over fifty-three or fifty-four weeks instead of fifty-two, but I was nervous about it nonetheless.

When 100 Pounds Down Isn't Enough

September 27, 2016
Tuesday Weight Report:
I have lost 4.0 lbs (four-point-zero) pounds since last week, putting me at 202.4 lbs, for a total weight loss of 103.2 pounds over 51 weeks. Since my goal was to reach 205.6, this puts me 3.2 lbs past my goal. My average weekly weight loss over the 51 weeks was 2.02 lbs.
I DID IT!
Well, it turned out the BMI said my weight should be between 147 and 179, so I decided to target 175, even though my doctor says the medical benefits of going lower than 195 are minuscule. Weight Watchers advises me to go for 175 but check myself, and seek outside opinion, every 5 lbs; that is what I am going to do.
I am also going to look into a slow-and-steady exercise program, like at a gym and stuff.
Thank you all for your continuing support through this! I'm going to continue to post these reports weekly even after the weight-loss part of my program ends, to help keep me on track. :)
EDITED TO NOTE: I still have the glam shoot coming, but it will have to wait until I recover from much intrusive oral dentistry and surgery. Thank you for your patience, please note.
Benchmarks Achieved:
100 pounds, 5 lb star, 100 lbs charm from WW.
"Glam" photo shoot in tailored suit.

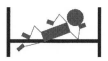

So I hit my target, which was wonderful. I had picked 100 pounds because it was a large round number and worked with the weeks in a year.

It didn't relate in any way to my health. It was time to check the real numbers.

One hundred pounds wasn't enough.

Using the Body Mass Index as my guide I would have to drop as least another twenty-five pounds and perhaps another fifty. I was advised to split the difference but check in every five pounds lost, which left me a bit at sea.

It was sort of like what C.S. Lewis said in *The Horse and His Boy*; I had learned that completing one difficult task led to having a harder one set for you.

I was used to knowing the precise amount of weight I needed to lose and tracking the time it would take me to get there. When I told my wife how much more Weight Watchers was saying I had to lose to make Lifetime it terrified her. I was already starting to be on the skinny side and enough was enough. We agreed I would see my doctor and follow his advice.

My doctor, having done a seat-of-the-pants (or rather, waist-of-the-pants) conversion from the height/weight ratio he prefers, determined that my optimum weight target would be 190 pounds, and that losing more than that would endanger my health rather than improving it. Weight Watchers accepted his note and reset my goal for Lifetime Membership to 190 pounds.

I had been so fat that losing "only" 100 pounds hadn't gotten me to a healthy weight. That threw me for a while.

I had to drop fifteen pounds more than I had expected. Annoying but, I hoped, doable.

Pain in the Mouth

October 4, 2016
Tuesday Weight Report:
I have lost 2.0 lbs (two-point-zero) pounds since last week, putting me at 200.4 lbs for a total weight loss of 105.2 pounds over 52 weeks. Since my goal was to reach 205.6 puts me 5.2 lbs past my original goal. My average weekly weight loss over the 52 weeks was 2.02 lbs.

My new goal is 190.0, with the following caveat:
The charts say my weight should be between 147 and 179, but my doctor has said the medical benefits of going lower than 195 are minuscule. Weight Watchers advises me to go for 175 but check myself, and seek outside opinion, every 5 lbs; my doctor said 190 so that is what I am doing.

I am slated for major oral surgery on Friday, Oct 14th, but after I recover from that, which should take about another six weeks, I am going to look into a slow-and-steady exercise program, like a gym and stuff.

Thank you all for your continuing support through this! I'm going to continue to post these reports weekly even after the weight-loss part of my program ends, to help keep me on track. :)

Benchmarks For Now:
< 200 Pounds for the first time since my mid-20s.
< = 195 Pounds Assess to see if continuing to lose weight is the healthiest option.
< = 190 FOR GOD'S SAKE STOP!

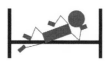

Graphic content warning: If details of oral surgery upset you, please skip to the next chapter.

I discovered a weird soft spot in the roof of my mouth. I went into my dentist, who took x-rays and determined that a one-inch square of bone in my palate was missing. He walked me down the block to an oral surgeon who said that yeah, it was missing alright, probably due to an infection that had gotten into the chamber between my mouth and nose and had been gnawing away at me for months.

Great. Just great. At least that explained the elevated level of calcium my doctor had found in my blood. It felt like an extremely poor reward for the hard work I had done on my health over the last year, and yes I did a whole lot of complaining about that. Over fifty, watching your health turns into a game of whack-a-mole. While you're fixing one issue something else pops up.

Turned out the fix for my condition was to drill a hole in my gums above the teeth, go in, clean up the infection, then essentially drywall the top of my mouth with cadaver bone then sew me up.

I complained a whole lot when this happened, and of course anything going wrong with my body just makes me want to eat more.

How Fat People See Me /When I See Fat People

October 11, 2016
Tuesday Weight Report:
I have lost 3.4 lbs (three-point-four) pounds since last week, putting me at 197.0 lbs, for a total weight loss of 108.6 pounds over 53 weeks. Since my goal was to reach 205.6 that puts me 8.6 lbs past my original goal. My average weekly weight loss over the 53 weeks is 2.04 lbs.

As I posted about earlier, I now fit nicely into size 38 pants classic fit; my starting point was size 52 stretch fit, which add about 2" to the size…:)
Benchmarks Achieved:
Less than 200 Pounds for the first time since my mid-20s.
Benchmarks for Now:
< = 195 Pounds Assess to see if continuing to lose weight is the healthiest option.
< = 190 FOR GOD'S SAKE STOP!

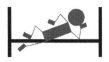

Now that I am among the thin, some of my friends who are fat, no matter how close we are, panic when they see me. It's as if my having lost weight means that I am now judging them like the rest of the world is, or that I will say "You could get thin too!"

I'm no longer on their team so they figure I am now the enemy. When I was fat it felt like the whole world had prejudged me and found me wanting. My friends now felt I would think of them the same way.

Am I pleased with myself for having pulled this off? Yes. I wouldn't be human if I weren't, or at least I wouldn't be me. Does that mean I have earned the right to be cruel to other people? No, it doesn't. No one has that right. So no, I don't look down on people who are fat, or simply having trouble with their weight. If they have made losing weight a priority in their lives, I'll help if I can, and if asked, and I will suggest they buy this book, but otherwise fat people have nothing to fear from me.

On the flip side, I've been asked if I see fat people differently now, no longer being one of them (although the future is always uncertain).

When I see fat people I see human beings who are muddling through life as best they can, just like I am. Who are looking for companionship, happiness, security, success, calmness and satisfaction just like I am. Who are as valuable to the world as I am.

Which is exactly what I saw before I lost weight.

A person's worth as a human being is not determined by dress size or collar size. No one's need to be loved is less than anyone else's, nor does how much they weigh determine their worthiness to be loved.

Pain In The Mouth Part II

October 18th, 2016
Tuesday Weight Report
Did not weigh in today due to simply being drugged, in pain, and wiped out. Hope to weigh in tomorrow, but may just skip it this week. Thanks, oral surgery!
Thanks to all those who cared enough to ask! Sorry no episode this week! :)
[My Facebook friends react to this news]:
Katharine Kroeber Damn! One of our favorite shows pre-empted for surgery!
Greg Cox What, we don't even get a rerun?
Shira Houghton Was thinking of you. Time to baby yourself for a bit.
John Ordover Greg Cox The show has been pre-empted for the premiere of the new show ORAL SURGERY: RECOVERY EDITION. I suppose I could post an update of that with bloody photos.
Katharine Kroeber No.
Heather Park-Albertson I've had to stop posting graphic images to my feed because the poor hubby can't handle in-your-face biology the way others in my family can.
Greg Cox I prefer the original series, not the grisly spin-off.
Susy Nerey Hope you are feeling better!
John Ordover More seriously, I did loosen the reins on my diet starting the week before; I still ate from the same selection of things, but I added a 10 AM and 3PM light snack. Still low-carb, low-fat.
Joe Mel Recover uneventfully and soon.
John Ordover OTOH, Greg Cox, perhaps every evening around 7 I will post an episode of TUESDAY WEIGHT REPORT: Year One. Hmm.

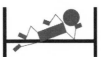

The oral surgery and the Really Good Drugs they had me on made weighing in more than I could handle that week. You'd think that pain-in-the-mouth would discourage me from eating, but it was just as hard not to eat as it had ever been. I was sleeping a lot though, and at least while I was sleeping I wasn't eating. I still did my best to stay with my plan.

To be clear I did not drop my diet for a week. I just cut myself a little slack.

I included the comments from my Facebook friends (with permission) because they were caring, amusing, supportive, and because it was part of why I thought about writing this book.

Skipping the Skip Week

October 25, 2016
Tuesday Weight Report:
I have gained 3.0 lbs (three-point-zero) pounds since two weeks ago, putting me at 200.0 lbs, for a total weight loss of 105.6 pounds over 55 weeks. Since my goal was to reach 205.6 puts me 5.6 lbs past my original goal. My average weekly weight loss over the 55 weeks is 2.01 lbs. My new goal is 175 pounds, with a stopover at 195. That gives me 5/25 pounds to go.

I still fit into size 38 pants classic fit, even if they are slightly snugger. :) My starting point was size 52 stretch fit, which add about 2" to the size....:)

I'm not surprised that I gained over the last two weeks, considering both pre-and-during-and-post surgical stuff, and advice from my surgeon, had me cutting back on portion restriction (although I kept the same limits on what kinds of things I ate). Plus being stoned on painkillers does not lead to good moment-to-moment decisions about food. :/

All in all, though, gaining 1.5 lbs per week for two weeks is something I know how to reverse and can jump right back into that, and also shows how, pun intended, thin the line between losing and gaining weight really is for me.

So, ONWARD!
Benchmarks For Now:
< = 195 Pounds. Assess to see if continuing to lose weight is the healthiest option.
< = 190 FOR GOD'S SAKE STOP!

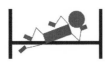

And that's what happened when I cut myself some slack on my diet. It taught me that the "skip days" and "skip weeks" that some diets push did not work for me. On my diet I lost weight; off it or even cutting it slack

I did not. To this day if I eat enough to not feel hungry, I gain weight rapidly. For me at least the only way to lose weight or even just keep my weight stable is to stick to an external plan under all circumstances. I wish it weren't that way but it is.

Back on Track

November 1 2016
Tuesday Weight Report:
I have lost 6.2 lbs (6.2) pounds since last week, putting me at 193.8 lbs for a total weight loss of 111.8 pounds over 56 weeks. Since my goal was to reach 205.6 puts me 11.2 lbs past my original goal. My average weekly weight loss over the 56 weeks is 2.00 lbs. My new goal is 175 pounds, with a stopover at 195. That gives me 23.2 pounds to go.

I'm not surprised that I lost so much over the last week, since I cut back down on portion control and carbs, having recovered from my surgery. Going up on carbs and on food means retaining more water, and last week's gain and this week's loss are related to that.

Benchmark Achieved:
195 Pounds Assess to see if continuing to lose weight is the healthiest option.
Benchmarks for Now:
< = 190 FOR GOD'S SAKE STOP!

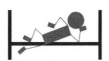

Back on my diet I was happy to have quickly lost the weight the two weeks off and the oral surgery had led me to put back on. I was no longer afraid of something happening that would make me put all the weight back on. I had locked in what I needed to do to lose it again, and more. It was comforting to discover I could turn things around so quickly, and that yes, much of what I had put on was water that dropped off as soon as I returned to my diet.

The End in Sight

November 8, 2016
Tuesday Weight Report:
I have lost 2.0 lbs (two-point-zero) pounds since last week, putting me at 191.8 lbs for a total weight loss of 113.8 pounds over 57 weeks. My average weight loss is just a smidgen under 2 lbs a week.

My doctor has told me that once I hit 190 lbs my best option, health-wise, is to stop losing weight and begin strengthening my core muscles, actually adding to my weight in the form of muscle. So my final goal is 190.0, which is 1.8 pounds away.

190 is the last Benchmark, and should be only a week so away at most.

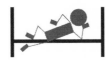

Since I had been told by my doctor that I needed to stop losing weight at 190 pounds, not 175, I was that much closer to my goal. It felt like I was cheating by moving the finish line, even though I knew that wasn't rational. The goal wasn't to hit a certain number; the goal was to get healthy. I accepted that 190 was my healthy weight and was certain I'd make it quickly.

Unwelcome Stability

November 15, 2016
Tuesday Weight Report:
I'm still at 191.8 this week, shooting for a doctor-mandated minimum of 190 lbs. So I didn't gain anything, but haven't moved closer to goal this week. My total weight loss remains at 113.8 lbs.

This week was at least a good lesson in what I have to eat and not eat to maintain a steady weight, and also a lesson in how, as your body mass drops, the line between losing vs. gaining becomes razor thin. One more helping of...well, anything, and I would have gained weight; one less helping of anything and I would have lost weight.

So, Onward to 190!

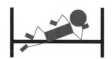

So of course I ran to weigh in that week in the hope that I would have crossed the finish line. Which I had not. But as I noted it did lead me to a greater understanding of what I needed to do to stabilize....

Bounce Back

November 22, 2016
Tuesday Weight Report:
I'm up 1.8 to 193.6 this week, shooting for a doctor-mandate minimum of 190 lbs. I think the flaw was that I have a nasty cold (which is fading) and I could not take being uncomfortable from both the cold and the eating plan. My total weight loss is currently at 112.0 lbs.

It also seems I have once again plateaued, which will require me to cut portion size once again, but not until next week, 'cause I'm not crazy.

So, Onward to 190!

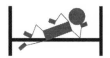

Or so I thought....

Back on Track II

November 29 2016
Tuesday Weight Report:
I'm down 1 lb to at 192.6 this week, shooting for a doctor-mandate minimum of 190 lbs (which as of today is officially recorded as my Weight Watchers goal for Lifetime Membership).

This weight drop, despite a not-at-all skimpy Thanksgiving Dinner, surprises and of course pleases me greatly!

So, Onward to 190!

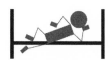

So back in the right direction despite hosting a holiday meal....

End Game

December 6, 2016
Tuesday Weight Report:
I made goal. I now weigh 189.8 pounds.
I'm down 2.6 lbs to at 189.8 this week, shooting for a doctor-mandated minimum of 190 lbs, which I have overshot a bit. Now I just have to figure out how to stay at this weight. I have no idea how to do that but I'll figure it out...

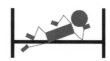

And then I was done. (See photo on next page)

Did this all add up to "doing next to nothing" like it says on the cover? In the sense that I did next to no exercise, yes. The rest adds up to changing what I was doing, not adding new things into my already busy, short-of-free-time life, and getting used to being uncomfortable a lot of the time. I know now exactly what I have to do to stay thin, and I know that it takes paying serious attention to everything I put in mouth and accepting annoying limits on my own behavior. So I am "embracing the suck" and staying on my current plan every minute of every day, which, as I said at the beginning, is an incredibly difficult thing. Wish me luck.

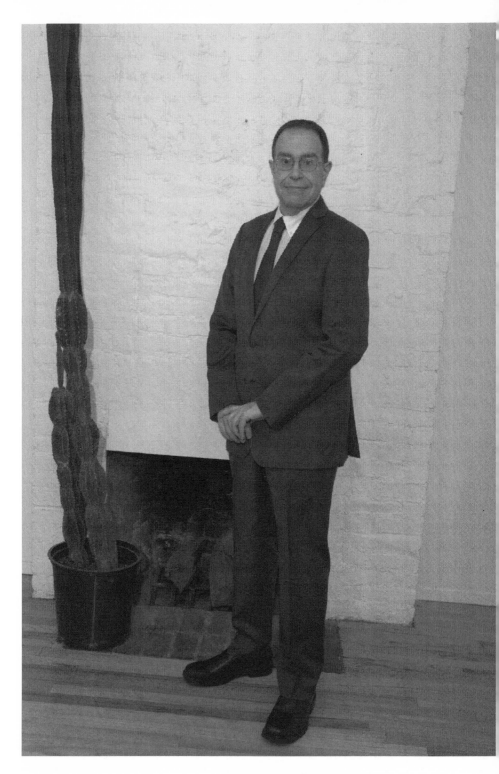

Afterword

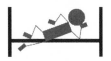

My diet is simple to lay out: I ate low-carb, low-but-not-no fat, low glycemic index food and I used strict portion control, which portions got smaller and smaller as I dropped body mass. I did not count calories, just limited my food choices to low-calorie foods. I avoided starchy foods like corn, potatoes, and carrots (dropped all tubers really), and limited fruit to berries, melons, plums, and nectarines (no citrus, no apples, no pears). I'm hypoglycemic so I was already avoiding sugar. I ate at 7:00 AM, 12 Noon, and 6:00 PM and did not eat between meals.

Cooking at home was, and is, delicious and varied, encompassing many cuisines, even under these restrictions.

A diet has to be right for the person doing it. This is what worked for me.

As of this writing it's been a year since I ended my diet, and I'm still hungry. That hasn't changed one bit. I'm still not exercising, although I'm looking for a way to work it so I don't wind up starving afterwards because I do think exercise will make me healthier.

I'm proud to say that my weight has pretty much remained stable. I'm usually within two pounds of 190 although whether I'm closer to 188 or closer to 192 varies, and I have gone over 192 from time to time.

I stay in that range by weighing in once a week no matter what, and if I go over 192 I reduce portions until I've evened out again. To take the pressure off I made a deal with myself: once I hit eighty-five years old, if my family is safely squared away, I will start eating freely again. Of course at that age I might well decide to push my Age Of Eating ahead to ninety-five.

My overall plan is to be healthier each birthday than I was the one before. I keep that up a couple of hundred years, I'm golden.

Acknowledgments

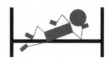

Heartfelt Thanks to:

Dr. Jonathon Brodie, Dr. David Case, and Dr. Susan Roberts, who provided much needed emotional support and/or medical advice at crucial junctures and without whom neither my weight loss nor this book would have been possible. Marv Wolfman without whose unwitting inspiration I might never have gotten interested in the mechanics of writing; Andy Richter who set me on the right path even though it wasn't the one he chose; Katharine Kroeber, who told me to be an editor in the first place and who provided constant support in tough times, both mine and hers; Carol Pinchefsky, for tossing me ideas when I got stuck; book designer Wrenn Simms, for taking on text organizational challenges that baffle me; Steven Barnes, and Karla Fisher whose wisdom, information and interest in my struggle was of great help even when I didn't agree with them; Kim Kindya and Nicholas Filip for their work on the iconography; David K. Randall for comradery-in-arms; Megan Randall for boundless enthusiasm unbowed by being surrounded by writers; Marilyn G. Ordover, my mother, for supporting me the whole way; my in-laws Dr. Paul Greenburg and Judy Greenburg, who got thin before me; and my Uncle Morris Ordover who was very pleased with my progress and who is sorely missed.

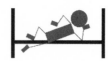

About the Author

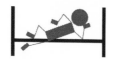

John J. Ordover is a noted editor, writer and troublemaker well-known for his work on the Star Trek novel line, for autism fundraising and for viral muckraking. He lives in Brooklyn, NY with his beautiful wife, special needs education advocate and political activist Carol Greenburg, and his handsome and athletic son Arren. Ordover has written television episodes and commercials, comic books and short-stories, and developed new marketing concepts while advising political campaigns and running fundraisers. Most days he can be found on Facebook, on twitter as @quotableordover and answering reader questions on his website lietherelosewight.com.

Made in the USA
Coppell, TX
17 January 2023

11245494R00092